Adult Transgender Care

Adult Transgender Care provides an overview of transgender health and offers a comprehensive approach to training mental health professionals in transgender care. The book takes an interdisciplinary approach to transgender care, emphasizing the complementary contributions of psychiatry, psychology, and social work in providing transgender care within an integrated treatment team. Included in this text are overviews of how to conceptualize and provide treatment with complex and difficult clinical presentations and considerations for understanding how to address system-level challenges to treatment. *Adult Transgender Care* meets a unique need by providing detailed information, clinical interventions, case studies, and resources for mental health professionals on transgender care.

Michael R. Kauth, PhD, is a clinical psychologist at the Michael E. DeBakey VA Medical Center in Houston, Texas, and one of two Directors of the Lesbian, Gay, Bisexual and Transgender (LGBT Health) Program within the Office of Patient Care Services in the Veterans Health Administration. Dr. Kauth is also co-director of the South Central Mental Illness Research, Education, and Clinical Center (MIRECC) and Professor of Psychiatry at Baylor College of Medicine in Houston.

Jillian C. Shipherd, PhD, is a clinical research psychologist at the Women's Health Sciences Division of the National Center for PTSD at VA Boston Healthcare System and one of two Directors of the LGBT Health Program within the Office of Patient Care Services in the Veterans Health Administration. Dr. Shipherd is also Associate Professor of Psychiatry at Boston University School of Medicine and is the author of over 80 peer-reviewed publications, many of which are on transgender issues.

Adult Transgender Care

[illegible]

[illegible]

[illegible]

Adult Transgender Care

An Interdisciplinary Approach for Training Mental Health Professionals

Edited by Michael R. Kauth and Jillian C. Shipherd

Routledge
Taylor & Francis Group
NEW YORK AND LONDON

First edition published 2018
by Routledge
711 Third Avenue, New York, NY 10017

and by Routledge
2 Park Square, Milton Park, Abingdon, Oxon, OX14 4RN

Routledge is an imprint of the Taylor & Francis Group, an informa business

Library of Congress Cataloging-in-Publication Data
Names: Kauth, Michael R., editor. | Shipherd, Jillian C., editor.
Title: Adult transgender care : an interdisciplinary approach for training mental health professionals / edited by Michael R. Kauth, Jillian C. Shipherd.
Description: First edition. | New York : Routledge, 2017. | Includes bibliographical references and index.
Identifiers: LCCN 2017026180 | ISBN 9781138229020 (hbk : alk. paper) | ISBN 9781138229037 (pbk : alk. paper) | ISBN 9781315390505 (ebk)
Subjects: | MESH: Health Services for Transgender Persons | Mental Health Services | Delivery of Health Care, Integrated | Patient Care Team | Transgender Persons—psychology | Adult | United States
Classification: LCC RC451.4.G39 | NLM WA 305 AA1 | DDC 362.2086/7—dc23
LC record available at https://lccn.loc.gov/2017026180

ISBN: 978-1-138-22902-0 (hbk)
ISBN: 978-1-138-22903-7 (pbk)
ISBN: 978-1-315-39050-5 (ebk)

Typeset in Bembo
by Keystroke, Neville Lodge, Tettenhall, Wolverhampton

Contents

Figures

Figures

[illegible] examin[illegible]
[illegible] relative to the [illegible]
[illegible] the [illegible]
[illegible]
[illegible]
[illegible]
[illegible] and geometric [illegible]
[illegible]
[illegible]
[illegible]
[illegible]
[illegible]

Tables

Contributors

Danielle S. Berke, PhD received her doctorate from the University of Georgia. She is currently a postdoctoral clinical research fellow at the VA Boston Healthcare System. Areas of interest include gender role socialization and psychological impairment, violence prevention, and trauma-informed psychotherapy.

John R. Blosnich, PhD, MPH is a research health scientist with the Center for Health Equity Research and Promotion with the U.S. Department of Veterans Affairs, VA Pittsburgh Healthcare System. His research areas of expertise include interpersonal and self-directed violence among lesbian, gay, bisexual, and transgender (LGBT) individuals with specific attention to suicidal risk and examining ways that social determinants of health can be integrated into adaptive health care systems.

Anne L. Boedecker, PhD is a licensed psychologist and senior gender specialist. She earned her PhD in Human Development at Pennsylvania State University. She has been in private practice in central New Hampshire since 1981, proudly serving the LGBTQQIA community. She now specializes in training and consultation with educators, mental health professionals, and the wider community. Dr. Boedecker is the author of *The Transgender Guidebook: Keys to a Successful Transition* and *The Transgender Workbook: Your Journey to Womanhood.*

George R. Brown, MD, DFAPA is Associate Chairman for Veterans Affairs and Professor of Psychiatry at East Tennessee State University. He served 12 years on active duty and 25 years in VHA, evaluating and treating active duty and Veteran transgender patients. Dr. Brown contributed to all versions of the VHA directive on transgender health care, has published extensively on transgender military/veteran issues, and has served 4 terms on the board of the World Professional Association for Transgender Health. He continues to provide training on transgender medicine for VHA and the Department of Defense.

Bryan N. Cochran, PhD is a Professor of Psychology at the University of Montana in Missoula. He is also a licensed psychologist and the Director of Clinical Training for the doctoral program in clinical psychology at the University of Montana. His research is focused on health disparities of LGBT individuals, particularly in the area of substance misuse.

Kelly Ducheny, PsyD is a licensed psychologist and Senior Director of Behavioral Health Services at Howard Brown Health Center, an LGBTQ Community Health Center. Dr. Ducheny completed a postdoctoral fellowship in integrated care at the Center for Healthy Communities at Wright State University and was a member of the American Psychological Association Task Force that developed the *Practice Guidelines for Working with Transgender and Gender Non-Conforming People*. Dr. Ducheny completed the Substance Abuse and Mental Health Services Administration-Health Resources and Services Administration's (SAMHSA-HRSA) Center for Integrated Health Solutions Health Disparities Leadership Program in 2012 and is the co-principal investigator on a HRSA Special Projects of National Significance grant exploring retention of transgender women of color in HIV care.

Anthony F. Firek, MS, MD is the Chief of the Section of Endocrinology at the Loma Linda VA Medical Center, a member of the VA National Transgender SCAN-ECHO and E-Consultation Program, and an Assistant Professor of Medicine at Loma Linda University of Medicine. Dr. Firek is a consultant Endocrinologist at the Riverside University Health System Medical Center affiliated with the University of California Riverside School of Medicine and is the director of the Clinical Research Group. His research interests include transgender medicine, development of vaccines for preventing diabetes mellitus, and thyroid cancer.

Hillary A. Gleason, MA is a fourth-year graduate student in the clinical psychology Ph.D. program at the University of Montana. Her research focuses on health disparities among LGBTQ and other marginalized populations, with a particular emphasis on providers' competencies.

Jamison Green, PhD, MFA is the immediate past-president of the World Professional Association for Transgender Health, author of *Becoming a Visible Man* (Vanderbilt University Press), and a policy consultant and transgender competency trainer for businesses, institutions and governmental agencies. He also provides expert testimony in employment discrimination litigation involving transgender workers. Additional information available at www.jamisongreen.com

Michael L. Hendricks, PhD, ABPP is a clinical psychologist in private practice at the Washington Psychological Center, P.C., in Washington, D.C. He is a fellow of the American Psychological Association (APA) and a past president of APA's Division 44, the Society for the Psychological Study of Lesbian, Gay, Bisexual, and Transgender Issues. He served on the APA Task Force that developed the *Guidelines for Psychological Practice* *with Transgender and Gender Nonconforming People*. He has conducted research with transgender and gender non-conforming people and is the lead author on the seminal paper on the minority stress model for transgender individuals. In 2015, he was awarded an APA Presidential Citation for his work. A primary focus of his clinical practice involves work with transgender and gender non-conforming adolescents and adults.

Ruben A. Hopwood, MDiv, PhD is the coordinator of the Transgender Health Program at Fenway Health since 2006 and a visiting researcher at The Danielsen Institute at Boston University. He earned his doctorate in Counseling Psychology and Religion from Boston University and has an extensive history working in mental health and social services in several states. In his work, Dr. Hopwood provides mental health evaluations, consultation, and clinical education on transgender health care. Dr. Hopwood is a published author in topics including transgender people in mental health, resiliency, religious, and spirituality issues.

Major Johnson, PsyD, ABPP is a licensed clinical psychologist and Major in the United States Air Force. Her research, policy, and clinical foci are lesbian, gay, bisexual, and transgender populations, Posttraumatic Stress Disorder, and mental health in veteran/active duty populations. She worked on the implementation of the Veterans Health Administration transgender veteran policy (2011) and the transgender open-service Department of Defense policy (2016). She is currently serving on active duty at Travis Air Force Base in California and has an appointment at the Edith Nourse Rogers Memorial Veterans Hospital, Bedford, MA.

Michael R. Kauth, PhD is one of two Directors for the LGBT Health Program for the Veterans Health Administration's (VHA) Office of Patient Care Services in Washington DC and has worked for the VHA for nearly 25 years. He also serves as Co-Director of the VHA South Central Mental Illness Research, Education and Clinical Center at the Michael E. DeBakey VA Medical Center in Houston, TX. Dr. Kauth is a Professor of Psychiatry and Behavioral Sciences at Baylor College of Medicine, where he teaches a course on LGBT Health. He has published more than 50 journal articles and 14 book chapters on topics that include health psychology, LGBT veteran health disparities, sexual health, implementation of educational interventions, and the evolution of human sexual attraction. Dr. Kauth is the author of *True Nature: A Theory of Sexual Attraction* (2000) and the editor of *Handbook of the Evolution of Human Sexuality* (2006).

Zander Keig, LCSW, MSW, MS is the Navy Medicine West Regional Transgender Care Team Clinical Case Manager at Naval Medical Center San Diego, CA and co-editor of *Letters for My Brothers: Transitional Wisdom in Retrospect* (Wilgefortis Press) and *Manning Up: Transsexual Men on Finding Brotherhood, Family & Themselves* (Transgress Press). He is also a clinical consultant, transgender competency trainer and National Association of Social Workers transgender subject matter expert. Additional information available at www.zanderkeig.net

Colt Keo-Meier, PhD is a licensed psychologist and medical student at the University of Texas Medical Branch in Galveston, Texas. He serves as an Instructor in the Psychology Department at the University of Houston, an Adjunct Instructor in Counseling at Southern Methodist University, and an Assistant Professor in Psychiatry at Baylor College of Medicine. Dr. Keo-Meier directs the Transgender Health Lab at the University of Houston, conducting research on the effects of testosterone on the mental health and sexuality of transgender men as well as the impact of parental support on the mental health of gender diverse children. He is a founder of Gender Infinity, a Houston-based organization created for transgender youth and their families in the South.

Alex S. Keuroghlian, MD, MPH is the Associate Director of Education and Training Programs at The Fenway Institute and the Public and Community Psychiatry Curriculum Director for the Massachusetts General Hospital (MGH)/McLean psychiatry residency program. Dr. Keuroghlian received his medical degree and Masters in Neurosciences from the Stanford University School of Medicine. He completed his psychiatry residency at the MGH/McLean Hospital training program, where he also served as Chief Resident in Public and Community Psychiatry. Dr. Keuroghlian was awarded the annual HMS Primary Clinical Experience Teaching Award by Harvard medical students. For two years, he was a Partners Healthcare Kraft Fellow in Community Health Leadership based at Fenway Health. Dr. Keuroghlian completed a Master of Public Health (Health Policy and Management) at the Harvard T.H. Chan School of Public Health. At Fenway, he works as a clinical psychiatrist within the Behavioral Health Department and also conducts research at The Fenway Institute.

Oakleigh M. Reed, BS earned his degree in psychology and sociology from Central Michigan University. Currently, he is a second-year clinical psychology doctoral student at the University of Montana. His primary research interests include analyzing motivations and impacts of anti-transgender prejudices and investigating barriers to care seeking among transgender individuals.

Joshua D. Safer, MS, FACP serves as the Medical Director of the Center for Transgender Medicine and Surgery at Boston Medical Center. He is also the Program Director for the Endocrinology Fellowship at Boston University Medical Center, the Director of Endocrinology Education at Boston University School of Medicine, and Associate Professor of Medicine at the Boston University School of Medicine.

Ranya Sawan-Garcia, PharmD is an ambulatory care clinical pharmacist specialist at the U.S. Department of Veterans Affairs (VA), Loma Linda and is the Lesbian, Gay, Bisexual, Transgender Veteran Care Coordinator (LGBT VCC) for the facility. She is a member of the VA National Transgender SCAN-ECHO and E-Consultation Program and is the senior lead pharmacist with transgender care team at the VA Loma Linda. Her areas of expertise and research interests include transgender medicine with emphasis on the pharmacodynamic and pharmacokinetic aspects of hormone therapy, development of local and national educational materials, and oversight of postdoctoral research projects involving transgender health.

Loren S. Schechter, MD is a plastic surgeon practicing in metropolitan Chicago and serves on the board of the World Professional Association for Transgender Health (WPATH). He received his medical degree, with honors, from the University of Chicago Pritzker School of Medicine and completed his residency in general and plastic surgery as well as a fellowship in reconstructive microsurgery at the University of Chicago Hospitals. While at the University of Chicago, Dr. Schechter was elected to the Alpha Omega Alpha honor society and graduated as The Outstanding Student in Surgery. Dr. Schechter was the local host for the 2007 meeting of the WPATH. In addition, he helped to author the 7th edition of the WPATH *Standards of Care*, and serves on the editorial board for two transgender medical journals. He authored the first surgical atlas, *Surgical Management of the Transgender Patient*.

Rebecca B. Schechter, MD is board-certified in Internal Medicine as well as Endocrinology, Diabetes, and Metabolism. She received her medical degree from the University of Pennsylvania School of Medicine and completed her residency and fellowship at the University of Chicago Hospitals. Most recently, Dr. Schechter was an Assistant Professor at the University of Chicago Medical Center.

Ladawn Sheffield, MA, LMHC is a mental health therapist specializing in transgender-affirming care in Portland, OR. She has previously worked at Fenway Health as a therapist and member of the Trans Health Team. Ms. Sheffield has a BSS in Comparative Religion from Cornell College and an MA in Counseling Psychology from Lewis & Clark College. She completed her clinical internship at the Sexual and Gender Minority Resource Center in Portland, OR and previously taught "Contemporary Issues in Transgender Studies" at the Experimental College at Tufts University.

Jillian C. Shipherd, PhD is one of two Directors for the LGBT Health Program for the Veterans Health Administration's (VHA) Office of Patient Care Services in Washington DC and has worked for the VHA for nearly 20 years. She is also a Clinical Research Psychologist at the

National Center for PTSD in the Women's Health Sciences Division where she studies gender differences in recovery from trauma. It is through this work that she began working with transgender veterans in 2001 and became passionate about health equality for LGBT veterans. As Chair of VA Boston Healthcare System's Diversity Committee, she passed the first local policy guaranteeing access to care for transgender veterans in 2007, which provided the foundation for the current national policy. She is also an Associate Professor of Psychiatry at Boston University School of Medicine and author of nearly 100 journal articles and book chapters on topics that include LGBT veteran health disparities, and the interface of mental and physical health in trauma recovery.

Colleen A. Sloan, PhD is a clinical psychologist at VA Boston Healthcare System and Assistant Professor of Psychiatry at Boston University School of Medicine. Dr. Sloan chairs the Interdisciplinary Transgender Treatment Team at VA Boston and serves as the psychologist team member of a national expert training and consultation team for transgender health in VA. Dr. Sloan provides direct clinical care, supervision, and education/training on Dialectical Behavior Therapy and LGBTQ health. She has published on topics of gender roles and LGBTQ health disparities, and she has developed significant interest regarding the utilization of evidence-based therapies for gender and sexual minority clients.

1 How to Begin

An Introduction to the Book

Michael R. Kauth, PhD
Jillian C. Shipherd, PhD

The views expressed in this material are those of the authors and do not reflect the official policy or position of the Department of Veterans Affairs or the U.S. Government.

Why write a book on adult transgender care for mental health professionals? The short answer—because there is a need to provide comprehensive information to mental health professionals who have been or will be providing care to transgender adults. There are good texts on transgender care for mental health professionals that discuss gender transitioning and mental health conditions, but these usually fail to discuss medical transitioning in sufficient detail and gloss over the mental health professional's role in collaborating and coordinating with prescribing practitioners and medical providers. There are also proscriptive texts for medical providers that focus on meeting the health care needs of transgender people, including medical transitioning, but these usually do not appreciate the idiosyncrasies of gender transitioning, or fail to address the various psychosocial needs of the transitioning person, or inadequately describe the critical role of mental health professionals. This book is different, in that it takes an interdisciplinary approach to adult transgender care that emphasizes the unique and complementary contributions of mental health (i.e., psychiatry, psychology, social work, and counseling) within an integrated primary care treatment team, or at least coordinating with a medical team. There are also important medical aspects of adult transgender care (e.g., hormone therapy, surgical interventions) that mental health professionals need to understand and take into account in their evaluations and in order to provide competent psychological care and support throughout the client's life course.

How many of you reading this text received any kind of training in transgender care in your graduate program? Probably very few, if any. This kind of content was not available when we were in graduate school. Not so long ago, graduate mental health professional programs viewed transgender people as curiosities—as something exotic—but also as a largely invisible population. There was no expectation that mental health professionals would routinely see transgender people in their clinical practice. And if one did see a transgender individual, the standard approach, not so long ago, was to focus on the individual's presenting problems of depressive or anxiety symptoms or relationship difficulties—and ignore any gender-related distress Gender dysphoria, when present, was viewed as peripheral. At the time, the prevailing view was that if the depression, anxiety, or relationship difficulties were well treated, then gender-related concerns would naturally resolve.

How can mental health professionals provide competent care if they ignore gender dysphoria—if they have little understanding of the phenomena of gender dysphoria, gender transitioning, or minority stress? Fortunately, in recent years, graduate mental health professional programs, as well as medical schools, have begun including content on transgender health and on the health of sexual minorities too. Professional training programs are beginning to respond to the increased visibility of lesbian, gay, bisexual, and transgender (LGBT) people in society and of people with various other sexual and gender minority identities that could fall under the LGBT umbrella (which we view inclusively). This book is intended to help new and established mental health professionals become better informed with and comfortable providing adult transgender care, especially within an integrated care team.

Another goal of this book is to help mental health professionals understand the necessity of educating support staff and clinical colleagues to create a welcoming clinic experience for transgender clients. Other disciplines besides mental health, such as internal medicine and endocrinology also tend to lack professional training in transgender care. Mental health professionals have an obligation to educate health care colleagues who are less knowledgeable about transgender care so that clients referred for services receive respectful, competent care. Training and education for support staff is also absolutely critical and often neglected. Transgender clients who have negative, demeaning experiences within the clinic environment—before they reach your office—are unlikely to hear what you have to say. Or ever return.

Like most established health care professionals who specialize in transgender health, we learned from experience—sometimes painful experience. In the process, we became educators about transgender health care. In 2011, when the United States Department of Veterans Affairs (VA) issued a national policy on transgender veteran care, we were asked to lead training for VA staff on the policy and its implementation. We leveraged that role into a formal LGBT Health Program within the VA Office of Patient Care Services, which put us in the position to educate the more than 305,000 clinical providers across 1,233 VA health care facilities on competent transgender care (VHA, 2016: www.va.gov/health/aboutvha.asp). Given the size of the VA health care system, educating clinical staff is an ongoing task. In an effort to expand clinical capacity for respectful competent transgender care in VA, we obtained resources to support training interdisciplinary treatment teams across the health care system using videoconferencing technology and case-based consultation by an expert team. At the time of publication, we will have trained 75 interdisciplinary teams and nearly 600 clinical providers through this tele-training/consultation program (Kauth, et al., 2015; Shipherd et al., 2016).

We have discussed with our colleagues in the U.S. Department of Defense how to implement this model for training among military health care providers, who have recently (as of June, 2016) changed their policies to allow openly transgender service members. A more detailed description of our efforts in VA is presented in Chapter 14. We produced this book in part to share our experience and knowledge in training multiple disciplines in integrated adult transgender care and improve care for the transgender clients we serve.

This book is intended as a self-guide for mental health professionals who want to become more knowledgeable about transgender care. This book may also be useful to medical providers who wish to have a better appreciation for the contribution of the other team members they work with in treating transgender clients. We have structured this volume to function as readings for, or the entire content of, a graduate-level mental health course on adult transgender care. We have asked contributing authors to present practical clinical advice based on best practices and to illustrate their content with case examples where appropriate. In addition, we have asked authors to include a short list of foundational readings at the end of each chapter. One essential recommended reading for this book—and not repeated in each chapter—is the World Professional Association for Transgender Health's (WPATH) *Standards of Care* (7th edition; 2011). The WPATH *Standards of Care* is a consensus document representing the minimum standard of practice for respectful, competent care of transgender people. All mental health professionals who work with transgender clients should be familiar with the WPATH *Standards of Care*, which provides guidance on gender counseling, conducting hormone and gender transitioning surgery evaluations, as well as how to write letters of support for name change or changing the sex listed on a client's birth certificate. Further, we strongly encourage readers to research their professional organization's policy position or code of ethics statement on working with transgender and/or LGBT clients. We have provided links to a few major mental health professional organizations at the end of this chapter.

The Words We Use

Readers who are even somewhat familiar with transgender issues will have noticed that language is important—finding a whole new vocabulary and sensitivity to language. Words matter. People are defined for better or worse by the words used to describe them or by the words they use to describe themselves. Words can exclude or include, control or liberate, demean or celebrate, make invisible or illuminate. Therefore, readers will find that contributors to this book have given great attention to language around transgender and gender non-conforming issues. However, language is also dynamic and evolving. The words we use today to replace outdated terms will themselves be replaced in the future. We will make mistakes and for that we apologize up front. For consistency and to show respect, we have made decisions about the language that we and contributing authors will use across chapters. For example, many terms are used to describe transgender and gender non-conforming people. The term "transgender" is employed in this volume as an umbrella term to describe a variety of presentations and a wide spectrum of gender identities. We intend this term to be inclusive of transgender-identified and gender non-conforming people, including those with non-binary identification. Some gender non-conforming clients will not identify as transgender persons. A general best practice is to reflect the words and labels that clients use to identify themselves.

Also, we view the term "transgender" as an adjective, as in "transgender men" or "transgender women," rather than as a noun. In this volume, authors for the most part will refer to "transgender men and women" rather than use the abbreviated "transmen" or "transwomen" which is less formal and more appropriate for casual conversation. We have avoided referring to "male-to-female" or "female-to-male" transgender individuals in favor of "transgender women" and "transgender men," respectively. We feel that referring to transgender people by their chosen gender identity, rather than by their sex assigned at birth, is respectful and a good model for mental health professionals. We have also avoided using the older clinical term "transsexual" unless it is employed for historical accuracy.

We recognize that not all gender non-conforming people identify with a transgender label. Some prefer terms such as trans*, non-binary, genderqueer, gender fluid, polygender, agender, and other identities. There is an ever-growing list of identity terms, but listing even some terms omits other possible terms. The client's preferred identity term should be the one used by health care professionals. However, given that language is evolving, we have chosen to use the umbrella term "transgender" inclusively, although it may not be the term your client prefers.

Throughout this book we primarily refer to "gender dysphoria" as a descriptive term for the distress that some transgender people experience. Our goal is to assist mental health providers in addressing this dysphoria utilizing an affirming framework. We sometimes refer to "Gender Dysphoria" which is a diagnosis in DSM-5 (American Psychiatric Association [APA], 2013) or "Gender Identity Disorder," which is an ICD-10 (World Health Organization , 1992) and DSM IV-TR (APA, 2000) diagnosis. Capitalization of these terms indicates that we are referring to a diagnosis.

We recognize that the goal of gender transitioning is to become more comfortable with one's physical body and gender presentation. The goal of gender transitioning is not necessarily to "change sex" or "become another sex" but rather to adopt a different gender role and identity from one's assigned sex at birth. Gender transitioning has no pre-determined end point, and the transition pathways are individualistic. In keeping with this non-binary gender, non-determinist view of gender transitioning, we refer to androgens as "masculinizing hormones" and estrogens as "feminizing hormones" rather than as "male hormones" and "female hormones," respectively. Of course, androgens are not exclusive to men, and estrogens are not exclusive to women.

Historically, gender transitioning surgeries have been referred to as "sex reassignment surgeries." We find that terminology outdated and inaccurate and use it only within historical context. We have encouraged authors to refer to "gender affirming" treatments, including "gender affirming surgeries," "gender transitioning surgeries," and even "transition-related surgeries."

By "mental health professionals or providers" we mean all mental health practitioners. There are a variety of mental health practitioners (e.g., psychologists, psychiatrists, social workers, counselors) who have distinct abilities, but here we focus mainly on the commonalities across mental health providers. We have tried to refer to specific kinds of mental health professionals only when referring to practices specific to those practitioners.

Because this text is focused on mental health professionals, we have adopted the less medical term "client" (rather than "patient") to refer to the people who receive treatment services. We have also taken an "interdisciplinary" treatment approach to transgender care that integrates various health care disciplines, including mental health, as part of a cohesive treatment team. We contrast this approach to a "multidisciplinary" model where various health care disciplines work independently and collaborate as needed but are not necessarily colleagues on an integrated care team. Of course, many readers will be working in a system that is more multidisciplinary in structure, but we encourage the application of an interdisciplinary model to care for transgender clients.

While we have attempted to produce a volume that is useful to mental health professionals in English-speaking countries, we readily acknowledge our cultural and national biases. We and the contributing authors are Americans, and we best know our own cultural experiences, even as we try to be conscious of cultural differences and health care system differences across English-speaking countries. Throughout this book, we have emphasized similarities across cultures as best we know them and have recognized differences where they occur. In addition, most chapter authors are cisgender individuals, although at least four authors identify as transgender people.

An Overview of the Chapters

This book is organized in 14 chapters. This first chapter provides context and lays out the major assumptions of the volume. In Chapter 2, Dr. Laura Johnson, a clinical psychologist and Major in the United States Air Force, gives a brief history of gender variant people and development of the contemporary conceptualization of transgender identities. Dr. Johnson describes how transgender people have been viewed and treated, mostly negatively, by various cultural institutions such as the military and organized sports. Mental health as a discipline has also played a major role in pathologizing transgender identities. It is critical for mental health professionals to recognize that unpleasant history and stigmatization by our profession in order to understand why transgender clients may be reluctant to talk with providers. Fortunately, all major mental health organizations are now supportive of respectful gender affirming treatments. That said, the controversial need to have a mental health diagnosis to access medical treatments creates a unique and complicated context for the therapeutic relationship.

Dr. John Blosnich, a public health researcher, discusses minority stress and intersectionality of identities in Chapter 3. Minority stress theory helps to explain how a stigmatized minority group, like transgender people, experiences health disparities compared to the general majority population. Minority groups within minority groups (e.g., African American transgender women) experience even greater health disparities. Dr. Blosnich describes this minority-within-minority or multiple minority status as an intersection of identities. He proposes a syndemic approach to care that attempts to account for the role that relationships between multiple identities have on health.

Chapter 4 focuses on creating a welcoming clinic environment for transgender clients. Here Dr. Bryan Cochran, a clinical psychologist, Ms. Oakleigh Reed, and Ms. Hillary Gleason, both psychology graduate students, set the stage for gender affirming care by presenting strategies for creating an affirming treatment setting. Simple suggestions include modifying intake forms for inclusiveness and posting signs or symbols that signify a warm and inviting environment for transition-related goals to be discussed. More difficult, but vital recommendations include examining one's own implicit biases about gender variance and directly addressing negative, transphobic remarks (e.g., in waiting areas, in therapy groups) when they arise.

The next five chapters each address specific treatment issues for gender dysphoria. In Chapter 5, Dr. Ruben Hopwood, a counseling psychologist, refutes the idea of a predetermined end point for gender transitioning. He describes various pathways that gender transitioning can take and offers a gender affirming approach to working with the client to identify their transitioning goals. Dr. Hopwood recommends that therapists work collaboratively with transgender clients to identify clear goals and discuss how these goals implicate other aspects of identity and functioning.

For those clients who pursue medical transitioning, Dr. Anthony Firek, an endocrinologist, and Dr. Ranya Sawan-Garcia, a pharmacist, describe the risks and benefits of masculinizing and feminizing hormone therapies in Chapter 6, with the mental health audience in mind. It is important for mental health professionals to understand masculinizing and feminizing hormone treatment options and their physiological effects to know whether a client's expectations are realistic and determine whether further education is necessary. This chapter provides easily accessible information, even for those who have not had medical training. This background will also help mental health professionals better communicate with medical professionals about treatment options and understand the health risks associated with hormone therapies.

In Chapter 7, Dr. Colleen Sloan, a clinical psychologist, and Dr. Joshua Safer, an endocrinologist and internist, discuss the management of high risk clients who wish to pursue gender transitioning. Unfortunately, as discussed earlier in this volume, some clients experience multiple and acute mental health conditions, such as severe depression and chronic suicidal ideation, or they lack social support, engage in risky sexual behavior, have an unstable living situation, or are homeless. Drs. Sloan and Safer offer strategies for reducing or managing multiple risks while continuing to pursue the client's goal to transition. The authors remind us that gender transitioning itself has emotionally stabilizing benefits.

In Chapter 8, Dr. Colleen Sloan and Dr. Danielle Berke, both clinical psychologists, go one step further by applying Dialectical Behavior Therapy (DBT) to address the emotion dysregulation that is common among high-risk clients. DBT has been used effectively to treat emotion dysregulation and extreme behavior that is often seen in individuals with Borderline Personality Disorder. Drs. Sloan and Berke note that the chronic invalidation of societies that devalue transgender identities may contribute to emotion regulation difficulties, impulsivity, and suicidality among transgender clients. They suggest that DBT can be a useful approach to keep clients engaged in treatment, lower risk behaviors, and develop effective emotion management skills in the service of transgender clients achieving their goals.

Wrapping up this section, in Chapter 9, Dr. Loren Schechter, a plastic surgeon, and Dr. Rebecca Schechter, an endocrinologist, describe the various surgical interventions encompassed in gender transitioning surgeries and the role of mental health professionals in evaluating and preparing transgender clients for surgical interventions. Drs. Schechter and Schechter emphasize the importance of good communication between the surgical center and the client's mental health provider. Their accessible descriptions of medical risks and complications of each procedure (as well as benefits) will be helpful to mental health professionals in making recommendations for gender affirming surgeries and to understand the recovery processes.

Aside from medical or surgical transitioning, transgender clients may need or request other interventions to support their successful social transition. For example, clients may need referrals for voice therapy, for example, to present as more feminine. In Chapter 10, Dr. Anne Boedecker, a clinical psychologist, portrays the mental health professional's role of coach in assisting the client in their gender presentation development. Transgender clients may need assistance finding transgender-friendly businesses for purchasing binders or packers as well as receiving help with hair styling, make-up, and clothing styles that fit and convey the image the client wants to project. Dr. Boedecker also notes the value of connecting transgender clients to community and peer support to further successful social transition.

Mental health professionals are often asked by transgender clients to provide support letters for change of name or change of sex on a birth certificate and other documents. In Chapter 11, Drs. Colt Keo-Meier, Kelly Ducheny, and Michael Hendricks, all clinical psychologists, outline the various support documents requested of mental health professionals and give examples. These authors note that requirements for changing official documents vary considerably by region and country, so it is important to know what is required in your locality. The authors also explain the value of "carry letters" and/or travel letters that may be requested to avoid harassment or unnecessary detainment by officials because the client's identity documents are not consistent with their appearance and preferred name and gender. In Chapter 12, Mr. Zander Keig, a licensed clinical social worker and active duty Navy service member, and Mr. Jamison Green, an attorney, outline strategies for finding additional resources for mental health professionals, such as website addresses for international and national transgender health organizations. Mr. Keig and Mr. Green also provide a helpful list of scientific journals that publish peer-reviewed articles on transgender health care.

Sexuality and sexual health are often neglected by health care professionals in general, due to personal discomfort or feeling poorly prepared to address these issues. Yet sexuality is an area of critical importance for most people, and no less so for transgender clients. In Chapter 13, Ms. Ladawn Sheffield, a Masters level counseling psychologist, and Dr. Alex Keuroghlian, a psychiatrist, discuss the role of gender within sexuality and describe ways in which sexuality and sexual relationships may change as a result of gender transitioning. They note that social transitioning, hormone therapy, and/or gender affirming surgeries can have profound effects on sexual attraction, libido, intimacy, and sexual functioning.

Lastly, we close this book with a chapter on implementing a transgender care policy within a national health care system. Drs. Jillian Shipherd and Michael Kauth, both clinical psychologists and editors of this book, and Dr. George Brown, a psychiatrist, briefly describe the implementation of a transgender health care policy for military veterans within the United States Veterans Health Administration (VHA) system as an example of how this has been done. We argue for starting with a clear health care policy as well as comprehensive patient and employee non-discrimination policies that include gender identity and expression. We also offer several lessons learned from our VHA experience that may benefit both large and small health care agencies as they consider their own transgender care policy.

In closing, the field of transgender health care is rapidly growing and inherently interdisciplinary. Both the rapid growth and interdisciplinary nature of transgender care represent significant challenges for the mental health professional, especially those who are new to this content. In this volume, we have attempted to provide an accessible body of knowledge to mental health professionals that will facilitate their collaboration with other health care professionals to provide respectful, competent care to transgender and other gender non-conforming people. Most mental health professionals reading this book may see only a few transgender clients in their practice. Our purpose is not to train specialists, although this book could be the start of such training. Rather, our aim is to help mental health professionals feel generally more comfortable and confident in treating the next transgender person who comes to their practice. Many of the necessary steps discussed in Chapter 4 advocate for making changes to your physical space, advertising, and intake forms even before you see your first transgender client. Ideally, this book is the start or a stepping stone in your pathway toward becoming more knowledgeable about transgender care. We also hope this volume will prompt mental health professionals to identify unintended barriers in their clinical practice and work to create a welcoming clinic environment for people of various gender identities.

National Professional Mental Health Organizations:

- American Psychological Association: www.apa.org/
- American Psychiatric Association: www.psychiatry.org/
- American Psychotherapy Association: www.americanpsychotherapy.com/
- (American) National Association of Social Workers: www.socialworkers.org/
- American Counseling Association: www.counseling.org/
- Australia and New Zealand Association of Psychotherapy: www.anzapweb.com/home.html
- Australian Association of Social Workers: https://www.aasw.asn.au/
- Australian Counselling Association: www.theaca.net.au/
- Australian Psychological Society: www.psychology.org.au/
- The Royal Australian and New Zealand College of Psychiatrists: https://www.ranzcp.org/Home.aspx
- British Association for Counselling and Psychotherapy: www.bacp.co.uk/
- The British Association of Social Workers: www.basw.co.uk/
- British Psychological Society: www1.bps.org.uk/
- (British) Royal College of Psychiatrists: www.rcpsych.ac.uk/
- Canadian Association of Social Workers: www.casw-acts.ca/
- Canadian Counselling and Psychotherapy Association: www.ccpa-accp.ca/
- Canadian Psychological Association: www.cpa.ca/
- Canadian Psychiatric Association: www.cpa-apc.org/
- European Association for Counselling: http://eac.eu.com/
- European Association for Psychotherapy: www.europsyche.org/
- European Federation of Psychologists' Associations: www.efpa.eu/
- European Psychiatric Association: www.europsy.net/
- International Federation of Social Workers: http://ifsw.org/europe/

Recommended Reading

Singh, A. A., & dickey, l. m. (Eds.). (2017). *Affirmative counseling and psychological practice with transgender and gender nonconforming clients.* Washington, DC: American Psychological Association.

World Professional Association for Transgender Health. (2011). *Standards of care for the health of transsexual, transgender and gender nonconforming people*, 7th edition. Retrieved from www.wpath.org

References

American Psychiatric Association. (2000). *Diagnostic and statistical manual of mental disorders* (4th edition), *text revision* (DSM-IV-TR).

American Psychiatric Association. (2013). *Diagnostic and statistical manual of mental disorders* (5th edition) (DSM-5).

Kauth, M. R., Shipherd, J. C., Lindsay, J. A., Kirsh, S., Knapp, H., & Matza, L. (2015). Teleconsultation and training of VA providers on transgender care: Implementation of a multisite hub system. *Telemedicine and E-health, 21*(12), 1012–1018.

Shipherd, J. C., Kauth, M. R., Firek, A. F., Garcia, R., Mejia, S., Laski, S. J., Walden, B., Perez-Padilla, S., Lindsay, J. A., Brown, G., Roybal, L., Keo-Meier, C., Knapp, H., Johnson, L., Reese, R. L., & Byne, W. (2016). Interdisciplinary transgender veteran care: Training for Veterans Health care Administration providers. *Transgender Health, 1*, 54–62.

Veterans Health Administration. (2016). *About VHA*. Retrieved from www.va.gov/health/aboutvha.asp

World Health Organization. (1992). *International statistical classification of diseases and related health problems, 10th revision* (ICD-10). Retrieved from www.who.int/classifications/icd/en/bluebook.pdf

World Professional Association for Transgender Health. (2011). *Standards of care for the health of transsexual, transgender and gender nonconforming people, 7th version*. Retrieved from www.wpath.org/

2 Scientific and Cultural Perspectives on the Gender Binary

Major Laura Johnson, PsyD, ABPP

The views expressed in this material are those of the author, and do not reflect the official policy or position of the U.S. Government, the Department of Defense, or the Department of the Air Force.

The concept of gender identity and the lives of gender variant people are in mainstream culture more now than ever before—with both positive images (e.g., transgender woman and American actress Laverne Cox on the cover of *Time* magazine) and negative portrayals (e.g., depiction of transgender women as predatory men seeking access to cisgender women and girls in public bathrooms). However, the multidirectional effect of transgender people, culture, and science predate both the modern progress of and backlash toward the transgender civil rights movement.

In North America, two-spirit and third-gender peoples within Native American and Indigenous communities predate the arrival of Western influence, though the term itself is more modern. Across tribes and languages in North America, more than 160 different traditions developed, including specific terms and local norms. Only in the more modern era (1990) have lesbian, gay, bisexual, and transgender (LGBT) Native peoples attempted to find language and community across those tribal divides (Pullin, 2014). A social justice movement has developed within Native American communities, both separate and distinct from, though undoubtedly influenced by, the transgender civil rights movement in broader society. Many in these communities see this movement as restoring two-spirit peoples to their original place of esteem in their Native communities, held before colonization, which brought new norms, values, and even forced assimilation (NativeOUT, n.d.).

Across the globe, there are other sociocultural ways of including gender variant communities. In Samoa, the *fa'afafine* (i.e., natal boys raised as girls but identifying as a third-gender) currently number around 3,000 (Abboud, 2013). As in other parts of the world, there is debate around whether one is born *fa'afafine* (i.e., the nature argument) or whether being raised that way to accommodate the needs of the family can sufficiently engender an adult female identity (i.e., the nurture argument). In South Asian culture, the *hijra* (neither male nor female identity) have widely varying roles across time, thought to bring luck to newborns, having served as royal bodyguards, and having a defined place in traditional Hindu culture. Currently, these revered roles are a thing of the past, and they suffer social ostracism and economic deprivation. They have recently won the right in India (2009) and Bangladesh (2014) to identify on official documents as a third-gender, and a Bangladeshi law was passed to work towards equality in education, employment, and social programs (Balbierz, 2014).

In modern America, Western Europe, and the United Kingdom (UK), transgender individuals are integrated into every area of life and industry, and are fighting for their civil rights. Though there are problems with prevalence estimates of this population, current estimates of the adult transgender population in the United States alone top 1.4 million (Hoffman, 2016); the prevalence in the UK is thought to be around 300,000 (Reed, Rhodes, Schofield, & Wylie, 2009); and in Western Europe there has been a three- to eight-fold increase in transgender individuals who present for transition-related care to gender clinics over the period covering the 1960s to 1990s (Zucker & Lawrence, 2009).

This chapter will: (1) explore transgender individuals' cultural place in the mainstream, as well as within subcultures from the 1950s onward; (2) review the medicalization of gender identity; and (3) identify the backlash to the modern transgender civil rights movement. In doing so, we hope to lay the foundation for a fuller understanding of how modern health care lays atop generations of oppression and exclusion, and that the role of health care equity is situated within a larger struggle for equality (Karasic, 2016).

Gender Identity and Mainstream Culture

Institutions

Western institutions have historically excluded individuals on the basis of sex. Certain professions, clubs, and franchises, etc. have only been available to men in the past. Various non-discrimination statutes, and even the 19th Amendment to the United States (U.S.) Constitution, have sought to remedy these areas of sex discrimination. Gender identity–based discrimination is a newer frontier—sometimes lumped into the *sex discrimination* category (as in the U.S. Affordable Care Act section 1557) and sometimes placed in a category of its own. We will look at two such institutions as they have grappled with inclusion: the military and organized sports.

The Military

The U.S. military is the newest in a list of nineteen countries that allows openly transgender service members. As the policy is new, the U.S. military has the opportunity to learn from the policies of the eighteen countries that came before (Australia, Austria, Belgium, Bolivia, Canada, Czech Republic,

Denmark, Estonia, Finland, France, Germany, Israel, the Netherlands, New Zealand, Norway, Spain, Sweden, and the United Kingdom (Elders, et al., 2014). The U.S. has a long history of transgender exclusion, despite documented transgender individuals serving honorably since at least the Civil War (Gansler, 2005) and an estimated 150,000 living transgender individuals serving or who have served in the military (Gates & Herman, 2014). Officially, transgender service members have only been allowed since a Department of Defense (DoD) policy change in June 2016, which impacts recruitment, retention, access to health care, and ability to serve openly. Prior to open service, studies with transgender veterans suggest that the experience of serving secretly due to an exclusion policy was a situation that too often led to harassment and violence (Harrison-Quintana & Herman, 2013).

This is a huge change for a military that until 2011 did not even allow open service of lesbian, gay, and bisexual individuals, and for its entire history has barred open transgender service. This exclusion has taken many forms (Witten, 2007), from barring admission through policy, discharging service members found to be transgender (with various discharge characterizations from dishonorable to honorable), and performing a medical exam upon entrance to the military to confirm sex (i.e., visual inspection of genitalia for purposes of determining birth sex and whether any genital surgeries have been performed). The change in policy to one allowing open service is an example of how large institutions are grappling with the reality of transgender identities and bodies.

Despite the progress that open service policies entail, the system is still a binary one (e.g., no process established for people who have non-binary identities), and as is generally the rule in the military, the transgender service member's commander has significant authority. According to the U.S. military's *Implementation Handbook* (U.S. DoD, 2016) for the open transgender service policy, commanders control timing of medical interventions (after consulting with military medical providers), have final approval over changing the member's gender marker in the personnel system, and throughout transition have the authority to allow or disallow exception to policy requests (e.g., a request to use bathrooms or lodging of their identified gender). Only once gender transition is deemed *complete* by the service member and their medical provider will the commander authorize a change in the gender marker in the personnel system that makes use of facilities, physical fitness requirements, and dress standards coincide with the service member's gender, rather than sex, a process which the handbook concedes can take more than three to four years. Notably, the handbook directs fellow service members that they each have a role in stopping bullying and harassment, using the Australian Air Force as a model for transition service members, and cautions military members not to "out" their colleagues.

The U.S. is only the most recent country to allow open transgender service. As noted earlier, at least eighteen other countries have trod this path before, with evidence that militaries can successfully integrate transgender service members, though none perfectly. Israel, which has compulsory military service, had historically excused transgender citizens from this duty under mental health exemptions. In 2013, the Israeli Defense Forces (IDF) first allowed a transgender female soldier to serve in the army. As they have integrated transgender service members into their forces, some report highly positive experiences and some report degradation and harassment (Schwartz, 2016). In order to provide more command guidance, the IDF renamed the Women's Affairs Department to the Gender Affairs Department. This department provides guidance for commanders with transgender soldiers, as well as guidance for transgender soldiers themselves. Additionally, Israeli military medical coverage includes cross-sex hormone treatments, although utilizing them can negatively affect one's career. Medical coverage does not yet include gender affirming surgeries (Schwartz, 2016).

While the U.S. and Israel are examples of nations that previously excluded gender variant prospective service members on the basis of a mental health condition, this was not the case in other countries. Spain's transgender exclusion had been based on medical exclusion—those who identified as male but lacked a penis and testes were medically excluded based on that absence. The Minister of Defence, responding to advocacy by a female-to-male prospective soldier, agreed to revise those medical exclusions in 2009 to allow for open service by transgender individuals (Pink News, 2009).

As militaries across the world begin to include transgender soldiers, sailors, and airmen, they are learning from one another's policies, mistakes, and corrections. The U.S. military's *Implementation Handbook* for transgender service members makes repeated reference to Australia's process, for instance. Evolution within an inclusion policy, like that described in Israel, will likely be the rule rather than the exception, as lived experience uncovers needs for each unique military structure.

Organized Sports

Sports have long been a gendered sphere of life. Cisgender male bodies are typically the norm, and the ideal, when a culture describes or represents athletes. Cisgender female athletes have had to fight this default conceptualization for as long as they have been involved in sports. In the U.S., Title IX legislation has sought to even the playing field since 1972 (Sinisi, 2012)—very recent in the span of human history. Sex parity was a goal, but this legislation failed to change the norm of sex segregation. Even where female athletes have made inroads—the Women's National Basketball Association (in the U.S.) or the Football Association Women's Super League (in the UK)—sports remain segregated. Part of the explanation for the status quo is that men's and women's bodies are inherently different. Intersex bodies question this narrative, and transgender bodies further complicate the easy, but inherently flawed, binary division. The view that human rights in sports is an essential sphere of consideration is beyond this chapter (see Kidd &

Donnelly, 2000), but organized sports are considered here as institutions within mainstream culture.

The Olympic Committee is perhaps the highest profile example of the struggle that mainstream institutions in the modern world have with incorporating transgender persons without wanting to upset the binary system of male/female categorization. Until the 2000 Olympic Games, the International Olympic Committee (IOC) could require a sex test (based on chromosomes) that was determinative of whether an athlete could participate in the selected sex category. Cisgender female athletes who were seen as too masculine and suspected of having a male sex have been subjected to sex verification testing, sometimes learning for their first time of an intersex condition (Padawer, 2016). The evolution of the IOC regulations from that point is illustrative of the changing nature of the mainstream understanding of transgender people.

In 2003, the IOC guidelines were updated to allow for transgender people to compete in the Olympics. This was partly due to a rising consensus that chromosome tests were no longer viewed as the whole story when it comes to sex. Medical guidelines to ensure "fair competition" (Associated Press [AP], 2016) were established. These guidelines required athletes competing in a gender other than their natal sex to have multiple medical interventions: gender affirming surgery, hormone treatment for a minimum of two years, and legal/governmental recognition of their gender.

In 2015, the IOC guidelines were updated to allow female-to-male athletes to compete without restriction in the men's categories (AP, 2016). Male-to-female athletes continue to compete under the requirements of medical intervention—documentation of one year of testosterone below 10 nanomoles per liter. A stated goal of these guidelines is to serve as a model for smaller international and national sports federations to follow, rather than encouraging a patchwork of regulations. One might argue that the IOC has evolved from seeing sex as a binary (based on XX or XY chromosomes), to seeing sex and gender as more complicated, whereas others will point to the continued forcing of all people—including gender variant people—to compete in a system with two categories: male and female. There were times when the IOC saw sex as requiring major medical interventions if an athlete competed in any but their assigned sex category. Presently the IOC only attempts to regulate the hormone that is believed to provide a competitive advantage—testosterone. This evolving view has led to more, though not complete, access for elite transgender athletes, though there were no out transgender athletes competing in the 2016 Olympics (Outsports, 2016).

Mainstream Cultural Depictions

Just as with large institutions, the representation of transgender people in popular culture has evolved. The earliest case of an out transgender individual becoming a media sensation is likely American Christine Jorgensen. She was a soldier in World War II, and following the war traveled to Denmark to have gender affirming surgery. She returned and held press interviews, had a nightclub act that went to Broadway, and told the story of her life through magazine, book, and film (Bilbrey, 2015). Ms. Jorgensen was a phenomenon—allowed by American society to tell her own story of transition and accepted as a woman, a picture of conventional femininity. Other transgender women in the early to mid-1900s, even those with access to gender affirming surgeries, hide their identities in public, as in the case of Lili Elbe (fictionalized in the film *The Danish Girl*) who pretended to be her own sister at times and faced rejection by friends and fellow artists who knew of her transgender identity (Harrod, 2016). Christine Jorgensen's story of acceptance is largely an outlier.

A far more common depiction from 20th-century America has been of transgender people as deranged, dangerous, or even murderous as in *The Silence of the Lambs* (1991). In this popular film, a transgender woman hunts cisgender women, keeping them in a hole and forcing them to soften their skin with lotion, for the purposes of murdering them, skinning them, and sewing together a new female skin for the killer to wear—a particularly grisly misrepresentation of transition. In another classic horror film, *Psycho* (1960), the killer cross-dresses as his dead mother. The deranged, evil transgender villain has been a steady theme of horror movies over the decades, as well as TV crime dramas (White, 2012).

The transgender villain role plays on cisgender people's fears of the unknown, cisgender people's comfort with the gender binary based on their own sense of gender matching sex (and concomitant discomfort with crossing the binary), and our human tendency to dehumanize those seen as *other*. Yet the reality is that transgender women, typically the section of the community represented as murderers, are much more likely to be victims of violence and murder. In 2014, 55% of U.S. hate-crime homicides within the lesbian, gay, bisexual, and transgender (LGBT) community were of transgender women (Ahmed & Jindasurat, 2015). Positive and more nuanced depictions of gender variant characters exist (e.g., *Ma Vie en Rose, The Crying Game, The Rocky Horror Picture Show*), but are often seen by more limited audiences.

There is a growing stream of media made by transgender people that incorporates their lived experiences or highlights transgender actors. These programs have begun to bring balance to the representation of transgender people in popular media—one of the only ways that the general population learns about the transgender community if they are not personally connected to an out transgender person.

Examples of positive popular media featuring transgender topics include reality television shows such as *I am Jazz* (2015–2016), *I Am Cait* (2015–2016), *Eurovision Song Contest* (1956–2016), and *Germany's Next Topmodel* (2006–2016), as well as scripted shows like *Orange Is the New Black* (2013–2016) and *Boy Meets Girl* (2014–2016).

In *I Am Jazz*, a reality show casts its lens on a transgender teenager. The main character, a transgender girl in Florida, was diagnosed with Gender Dysphoria at age four and began her social transition at age five. In 2006, she was interviewed for television and has remained in the spotlight ever since. The reality show portrays many aspects of one transgender girl's life—from dealing with transphobia, to the complexities of dating, to aspects of physical transition. It is a venue in which a transgender person's story is told, in part, through her own words, and those of her family's. Although not the typical story of a transgender teenager, this show brings an actual transgender person into the living rooms of its viewers, sharing her life and its human challenges. *I Am Cait* is Caitlyn Jenner's reality television show where she publicly discusses life as a transgender woman, often inviting transgender activists to participate, such as Kate Bornstein, Mara Keisling, and Candis Cane. Caitlyn is well known in America as former Olympian Bruce Jenner as well as for being a parent and participant on *Keeping Up with the Kardashians*. In *Germany's Next Topmodel*, the 2015 cycle of the show featured a transgender female participant. She is of Iranian descent, raised in the Netherlands, and has had to fend off reporters' intrusive questions about her history of surgeries and the current state of her bodily transition. Like other transgender celebrities, she has rebuffed these attempts. *Eurovision*, which has been a mainstay in Europe for over 60 years, has had two transfeminine performers win in its history. In 1998, Dana International, an Israeli transgender woman won the competition, and in 2014, Conchita Wurst (an Austrian performer, who self describes as a "man in a dress"; McCormick, 2015) won.

Orange Is the New Black (2013-2016) is a show primarily about a cisgender woman who is incarcerated in a women's prison. In the prison, a transgender character (Sophia Burset, played by Laverne Cox, a transgender woman) is fleshed out over several episodes. During her incarceration, Sophia is placed in solitary confinement following an anti-transgender assault; the prison leadership rationalizes that because they cannot keep her safe from violence in the general population then solitary placement is the best solution. Sophia is shown to be a parent, a spouse, and an entrepreneur. Despite this progress, a transgender character being played by a transgender actress is quite rare (Bilbrey, 2015).

In 2013, the British Broadcasting Corporation (BBC) staged a contest (*Trans Comedy Award*) to find good scripts with positive portrayals of transgender characters. *Boy Meets Girl* (2014–2016) was the result and has so far been commissioned for two seasons. The series is a romantic comedy about a 26-year-old man and 40-year-old woman who begin dating. The main female character is a transgender woman and is portrayed by a transgender actress. One series subplot focuses on physical intimacy in a cisgender/transgender relationship and another focuses on the way that transgender women can be targets of inappropriate attention from society and cisgender men in particular. In the second series of the show, a transgender male character is introduced (Charlie), played by British actor and transgender man Tyler Luke Cunningham. The two characters meet in a transgender support group. Both actors are able to bring their lived experience of transitioning to the roles (Cox, 2016).

One thing these pieces of popular culture have in common is that they all depict transgender women or transfeminine gender variance. This may reflect the media's continued fascination with transgender women over transgender men and those who have non-binary identifications, with the notable exception of *Boys Don't Cry*, a 1999 film about the real-life murder of a transgender man. Many media portrayals of transgender women focus a significant amount of attention on their bodies—showing them putting on makeup or female clothing items. As with cisgender women, transgender women's bodies are objectified in the mainstream culture.

Lesbian, Gay, and Bisexual Communities

Although the acronym LGBT suggests one big community, the included communities have not always seen their struggles as similar (Mottet & Tanis, 2008). The LGBT acronym collapses multiple realities—same-gender or multiple gender sexual attraction, and gender variance—into one category. In reality, sexual orientation and gender identity are orthogonal characteristics. A transgender person may identify as straight, gay/lesbian, bisexual, or queer. A gay person may identify as cisgender, transgender, or genderqueer.

LGB organizations have had various levels of welcoming transgender individuals over the years—ranging from complete exclusion to complete inclusion. It is important to remember that gay and lesbian organizations were themselves typically separate at the start of the American lesbian and gay rights revolution; the 1950s saw the founding of the Mattachine Society for men and the Daughters of Bilitis for women. Later in the movement, bisexuals began to fight for representation and inclusion in community events like pride parades; a fight for inclusion still continues (Milliken, 2014). Although the (sometimes uneasy) alliance between the L, G, and B communities is commonplace at this point, transgender inclusion remains challenging.

The Daughters of Bilitis, an American lesbian civil rights organization founded in 1955, kicked out a transgender woman in 1972 because they did not recognize her as female (Bilbrey, 2015). Examples of more recent exclusion can be found at the Michigan Womyn's Music Festival (MWMF), which was established in 1976 as a women-only, lesbian-feminist event where women could be free of patriarchy and fear. In 1991, the MWMF forced a transgender woman to leave and enacted a policy stating that the festival is only for "womyn-born-womyn". Transgender women and their allies held an annual parallel demonstration starting in the 1990s outside MWMF, called Camp Trans. Many artists boycotted the MWMF for its exclusionary policy, which perhaps led to the end of the 40-year-old festival in 2015.

Other organizations provide examples of evolution to full inclusion. The Gay City Health Project in Seattle, WA started as an organization for gay men growing out of the AIDS crisis and subsequently evolved to fully include transgender men by name in all of its events, publications, and mission (Mottet & Tanis, 2008). Most Pride parades and Christopher Street Days

(European pride celebrations celebrated around the anniversary of the Stonewall riots) across the U.S. and Europe include transgender pride as part of their mission. Some cities even have additional events focused on transgender pride, such as San Francisco's Trans March or the Trans Pride South West in Bristol, UK. Individual LGBT organizations continue to have varying levels of transgender inclusion, although the trend is for more, and better thought-out, inclusion—in language, resources, and policy.

The discomfort of proximity for these communities can run both ways. Well-known transgender individuals have publicly expressed negative feelings towards the LGB community. Christine Jorgensen, who famously transitioned in the 1950s, considered "homosexuality as immoral" (Bilbrey, 2015). Much more recently, American Caitlyn Jenner, who transitioned in the 2010s, expressed lack of support for same-sex marriage rights. Though there is significant public pressure for LGBT communities to act as one, as with any community, heterogeneity far exceeds homogeneity.

Laws and Policies

As of 2016, eighteen of fifty states in the U.S. had laws protecting transgender individuals from discrimination in public accommodations. This is an evolution from the start of the transgender civil rights movement, which can be traced back to the San Francisco Compton Cafeteria riots of 1966 and the New York City Stonewall riots of 1969, both protesting police harassment. At that time, transgender people routinely faced police harassment and arrest in public spaces. They had no legal protection from discrimination (e.g., housing, employment), and basic rights—like changing one's name—were denied. In the face of discrimination and violence, members of gender variant communities fought back physically, through riots, and socially, through political activism. In 1975, Minneapolis, MN passed the first known U.S. law protecting transgender individuals. Since that time, activism has come in waves, spurred forward in the aftermath of hate crimes, civil rights issues, and via community building during and following the initial AIDS epidemic (Stryker, 2004).

The global evolution of allowing official designations beyond the gender binary is ongoing. In the 1970s, Sweden became the first country to allow a change in sex designation on legal documents. In 2009, both India and Pakistan allowed for gender markers other than male and female on national identification cards. In 2003, Australian birth certificates could indicate an "X" for indeterminate birth sex and in 2011 passports could also indicate an "X" for indeterminate gender. In 2013, Germany became the first European country to include an indeterminate designation ("X") on birth certificates. A French court recognized a "neutral gender" category in 2015, but this ruling was reversed on appeal. Germany's high court also struck down the indeterminate designation in 2016, reasoning that the legal right since 2013 to leave the sex entry blank on birth registries fulfills the rights of the German intersex community and that a separate sex designation is unnecessary (Shalal, 2016).

Currently, transgender civil rights remain a patchwork across the U.S. The U.S. Transgender Survey (James, Herman, Rankin, Keisling, & Ana, 2016) paints a grim picture. Hate crimes and murders among the transgender population remain high, as do suicide attempts within the community (40%). Poverty can be extreme in this population, with transgender people of color being hardest hit. Transgender children are facing harassment and victimization in schools, both from peers and from teachers and administrators. U.S. federal action supporting bathroom use based on gender identity in schools was a hopeful sign, though was reversed in 2017, and a positive lower court ruling (*Gloucester County School Board v. G. G.*) is currently on the Supreme Court docket for review (n.d.). Discrimination in employment affected many of those surveyed, with 16% directly losing their jobs due to gender identity (James et al., 2016). In the U.S. there remains no national antidiscrimination employment law for transgender people. High rates of homelessness in the past year (12%) due to gender identity correspond with other negative outcomes—including harassment and assault at shelters. There remain significant barriers to health care, including insurance policies not covering transition, physician bias and ignorance of transgender health care needs, and HIV infection rates five times the general population. For those who have transitioned, only 11% reported being able to update all their identity documents to reflect their appropriate gender. Police harassment—the catalyst of the modern gay and transgender rights movements—remains high for transgender individuals, with 58% of survey respondents who had interacted with police in the past year reporting mistreatment. Physical assault and sexual assault for incarcerated transgender people also remains high (23% and 20%, respectively). Despite increased cultural visibility, the day-to-day life of transgender people remains affected by discrimination and violence.

A similar patchwork exists across Europe. Thirteen countries outlaw transphobic violence specifically (hate crime laws; Transgender Europe, 2016). Twenty-two countries offer legal protection from employment discrimination, and European Union (EU) law and the European Court of Human Rights provide anti-discrimination protections. Forty-one European countries offer some kind of official legal recognition of changed gender, though twenty-three of those (including thirteen in the EU) require sterilization prior to legal recognition. However, three countries cover transgender non-discrimination in their constitutions (Austria, Malta, and the UK; Transgender Europe, 2016).

Medicalization of Gender Identity

Psychiatry and the Diagnostic and Statistical Manual (DSM) of Mental Disorders

Psychiatry has been involved in the medicalization of gender identity since its modern inception. Richard von Krafft-Ebing's study *Psychopathia Sexualis* (1894/2012) was written with the specific intention of addressing physicians and excluding the public from his discourse on sexuality and gender. Early work on gender variance by the medical and mental health professions was primarily pathologizing. Gender variance was seen as a mental problem, whether identifying the problem's location in biology or in childhood upbringing (Cauldwell, 2006). In the early 1920s, prior even to a modern understanding of the relationship of hormones to gender expression, the first known gender affirming surgery (male-to-female) was performed at the Hirschfeld's Institute for Sexual Science (prior to its destruction by the Nazis; Beemyn, 2014). In the following decade, the first medical doctor used hormones (in addition to surgeries) as part of gender transition (female-to-male; Pelleschi, 2016).

By 1952, the American Psychiatric Association (APA) sought to establish a comprehensive nomenclature for psychiatric disorders, as at the time there were multiple nomenclatures at work in the U.S. alone. In the original *Diagnostic and Statistical Manual of Mental Disorders* (DSM-I, APA, 1952), gender variance along with homosexuality and pedophilia were referenced under the diagnosis of Sexual Deviation (transvestism). This classification continued in DSM-II (APA, 1968). By DSM-III (APA, 1980), Gender Identity Disorder (GID) was codified. While identifying the disorder within the individual, DSM-III educated providers on the distinctions between various terms related to gender: sex, gender identity, gender role, and expectations associated with gender role. DSM-III also separated GID from paraphilias (e.g., transvestism). DSM-IV (APA, 2000) continued the diagnosis of GID.

Much controversy surrounded the writing of DSM-5 (APA, 2013) and the creation of Gender Dysphoria as a diagnosis. Transgender advocates were not uniform on the diagnosis issue—some advocated for total removal of transgender-related diagnoses from DSM-5, arguing that inclusion was stigmatizing of an identity and did not contribute to the well-being of the transgender community. The parallel was made to homosexuality—a diagnosis that was eventually removed after years of activism both within APA by psychiatrists themselves and from outside the organization by gay rights activists. Advocates argued that just as homosexuality was removed because the field now recognizes gays, lesbians, and bisexuals as not inherently disordered, so should gender diagnoses be removed as an acknowledgement that transgender individuals are not inherently disordered.

Other professional and transgender community advocates disagreed. Transgender individuals are in the somewhat unique position medically of needing access to medical services (e.g., cross-sex hormones, gender affirming surgeries) as part of a physical transition based on an identity variable (though it should be noted that not all gender variant people choose medical interventions to transition, and others do not have access to transition-related medical services). Physicians, surgeons, and other health care providers need a diagnosis to justify provision of services as medically necessary rather than purely cosmetic. Therefore, some advocates argued for keeping a diagnosis related to gender dysphoria (allowing treatment of distress, rather than identity) to maintain access to needed health care services.

Ultimately, this was the change made in DSM-5 (2013). Gender Dysphoria (GD) was created and given its own category. The text no longer locates the disorder within the identity itself but re-locates it in the distress associated with the conflict between birth sex and gender identity, which assumes that there are transgender individuals without distress who would not meet criteria for the diagnosis. The text also specifically identifies the spectrum of gender variance existing outside the binary, acknowledging that a binary conceptualization is not necessary to treat gender dysphoria. Thus, the GD diagnosis allows medical and mental health care providers to code encounters, although some advocates continue to argue that a diagnosis inherently stigmatizes the gender variant community and locates the disorder within them, rather than within the society that presents the individual with oppression and often violence.

The International Classification of Diseases (ICD)

In contrast to the DSM, the International Classification of Diseases (ICD) began as a nosology of medical disorders. It was not until the sixth edition that mental health disorders were even included, and no diagnosis related to gender variance was included at that time (Drescher, 2016). Transsexualism was added three editions later, in the mid-1970s, in the mental and behavioral disorders section (rather than the medical health section) of the classification system. The ICD-10, issued in 1992 (with a clinical modification in 2016) switched to Gender Identity Disorder (GID) in childhood or adolescence or in adulthood (World Health Organization, 1992). The ICD-11, expected to be published in 2018, will move the gender variance diagnosis out of the mental health section of the codebook and into the physical health section, with a name change to Gender Incongruence (Belluck, 2016). Theoretically this change will allow Gender Incongruence to be part of the sexual health section and will provide an affirmative response to the United Nations member states, including the European Parliament, who have asked for this change (Reed et al., 2016). In addition, moving gender variance out of the mental health section suggests that psychiatric specialists are not required for care, which has created barriers to receiving care; insurers have routinely barred transition-related coverage, perhaps in part because it has been seen as psychiatric and not medical. Removal of a gender variance diagnosis altogether will add different barriers relative to insurance, so retention of a diagnosis in ICD-11 may be appropriate given the current medical systems in place across the world.

A field study of transgender-identified people in Mexico found that although a majority of transgender individuals retrospectively report a high level of distress in adolescence, this experience is not universal (Robles et al., 2016). Regression analyses pointed to social rejection as the single largest predictor of distress and impairment among participants, which belies the idea that distress is an inherent feature of gender incongruence, rather than a response to social oppression. These results were cheered by transgender groups such as Global Action for Trans* Equality.

International Standards of Care

Harry Benjamin was a German-born endocrinologist/sexologist who began practicing in the U.S. in 1914. He was a pioneer of what are now known as affirmative therapies—treatments for gender dysphoria that focus on changing the individual's gender rather than forcing them to accept their sex assigned at birth. Using cross-sex hormone treatment and working with clients to access surgeries, Dr. Benjamin became well known for his work with the transgender community.

An organization devoted to transgender health was named after him upon its creation in 1979: the Harry Benjamin International Gender Dysphoria Association. It published its first *Standards of Care for the Health of Transsexual, Transgender, and Gender Nonconforming People* in that year, advocating for a standardized and affirmative approach to the treatment of transgender individuals seeking medical interventions related to transition. The organization, since renamed the World Professional Association of Transgender Health (WPATH), is on its seventh version of the *Standards of Care* (available in twelve languages) and publishes a peer-reviewed journal (*International Journal of Transgenderism*). Although mental health care is included in the *Standards of Care*, it is one of several specialties addressed, including endocrinology, reproductive health, voice and communication therapy, surgery, and primary care. The focus of the *Standards of Care* is not to pathologize, or to locate a problem, but to "promote evidence-based care" (WPATH, 2011).

In the U.S., the WPATH *Standards of Care* are not codified as official treatment guidelines. However, the Affordable Care Act, Section 1557, has been interpreted by the Department of Health and Human Services (DHHS) as providing protection for transgender individuals from discrimination in their health care (DHHS, 2016). The WPATH *Standards of Care* give health care providers a model for how to provide gender affirming care with gender non-conforming populations.

Scientific Understanding on Origins of Transgender Identity

Initially, gender-identity theorizing was located in psychodynamic thought (Stoller, 2006), followed by learning theory (Money, Hampson, & Hampson, 1957). More recently, scientists have turned to more biological origins—namely, neuroanatomical differences. Differences have shown up in individual studies; the following are areas where the brains of transgender individuals better match identified gender compared to the natal sex group: white matter fiber structure, gray matter in the putamen (right hemisphere), the bed nucleus of the stria terminalis, the third interstitial nucleus of the anterior hypothalamus, and cortical thickness (Luders et al., 2012). There are several problems with interpreting findings from these studies—notably, the use of cross-sex hormones is a confounding variable, along with small sample sizes, treating all male-to-female or female-to-male transgender individuals as a homogenous group, and the use of post-mortem brains. Other studies have found no differences between transgender brains and the neuroanatomy of matched natal sex cisgender controls (e.g., Emory, Williams, Cole, Amparo, & Meyer, 1991).

Another biological theory comes from drug research. Diethylstilbestrol (DES) is a synthetic hormone that was prescribed to pregnant women for decades (1940s–1970) before being discontinued due to increased cancer risk for the children of those pregnancies. Retrospective studies on samples of affected children have found a 50% rate of identifying as transsexual or transgender, although more research needs to be done (Rudacille, 2005). This finding suggests that estrogens/synthetic estrogens may play a role in utero on postnatal gender identity.

Backlash

The gains of transgender rights and representation, although far from completely realized, are facing backlash in the 2010s. One marker of backlash is the high rate of violence against transgender individuals (Michaelson, 2015). Internationally, activists and community members annually recognize Transgender Day of Remembrance, a day to honor gender variant murder victims around the globe. The event began in 1999 following the murder in Massachusetts of transgender woman Rita Hester; it is placed in November, the month of her murder (Abernathy, 2007), and has spread across the world. Remembrances often consist of a candlelight vigil and a reading of the names of the known victims; they serve to raise public awareness of the violence against the transgender community.

Another marker of backlash is a spate of proposed laws in the U.S. prohibiting transgender individuals from using the public bathroom consistent with their gender. Some states, like North Carolina, have even restricted cities from passing anti-discrimination laws aimed at protecting gender non-conforming people. The loss of legal rights and the depiction of transgender people (typically transgender women) in these arguments as men who are attempting to gain access to female spaces in order to victimize cisgender women and girls are damaging in and of themselves. State politicians and the U.S. federal government are at odds in this area, with the U.S. Department of Education and Department of Justice directing public schools to provide a non-discriminating environment for transgender students (e.g., bathrooms, athletics, privacy, records) backed with the weight of potential funding cuts. However, state politicians, religious activists, and many cisgender Americans publicly oppose this move as government over-reach and an imposition of values without local input (Sanchez, 2016). The EU has also come out against discriminatory U.S. laws, pointing to the International Covenant on Civil and Political Rights, a United Nations resolution to which the U.S. is a signatory (EU Spokesperson, 2016).

Public backlash is not restricted to federal governmental policies or state laws. When a major American big box store, Target, publicly announced that it would allow customers and employees to use bathrooms consistent with their gender (versus their sex assigned at birth), a consumer boycott reportedly cost the brand over one million shoppers (Zaimov, 2016).

Despite the backlash, U.S. legal scholars argue that the overall thrust of legal and policy victories has been advantageous for the LGBT communities as a whole (Keck, 2009). In Europe, there is hope that as states join the EU, they will adopt its view of LGBT human rights. This has not been uniformly true, particularly in Central European countries, and there are no specific measures for the EU to change the attitudes of these other states (Csaky, 2014).

Take Home Points

- Gender variant people predate modern countries and concepts of gender and the binary (and its deconstruction) continue to evolve.
- Mainstream institutions have historically excluded transgender individuals (e.g., military, organized sports), but this practice is changing as advocates exert pressure on these institutions.
- Cultural depictions of transgender individuals are historically negative, but as transgender people become involved in the creation and depiction of these portrayals the landscape is becoming more positive and more nuanced.
- Transgender individuals continue to face oppression and exclusion from broader society as well as from the lesbian, gay, and bisexual communities.
- The transgender civil rights movement has seen significant progress but also significant backlash; gender variant individuals remain at increased risk for physical, emotional, and sexual violence, suicide, and discrimination in employment and housing.
- Psychiatry and medical professionals more broadly have medicalized gender variance in ways both negative (e.g., pathologizing) and potentially positive (e.g., creating pathways to medical transition). Transgender affirmative care is more common now, although not necessarily widespread. Recognized standards of care exist to guide treatment.

Suggested Viewing

Davis, K. (Producer & Director). (2001). *Southern Comfort* [Motion Picture]. United States: HBO Documentary.

Livingston, J. (Producer & Director). (1991). *Paris is Burning* [Motion Picture]. United States: Miramax Films.

Silverman, V., Stryker, S., & Walsh, J. (Producers) & Silverman, V. & Stryker, S., (Directors). (2005). *Screaming Queens: The Riot at Compton's Cafeteria* [Motion Picture]. United States: Frameline.

References

Abboud, P. (2013, July 16). Fa'afafine: The boys raised to be girls. *Special Broadcasting Service*. Retrieved from www.sbs.com.au/news/article/2013/07/16/faafafine-boys-raised-be-girls

Abernathy, M. (2007). About TDOR. In *International Transgender Day of Remembrance.* Retrieved from https://tdor.info

Aengus, J., Miller, C. K., & St. John, D. (Producers). (2015–2016). *I am Jazz* [Television Series]. Silver Spring, MD: TLC.

Ahmed, O., & Jindasurat, C. (2015). *Lesbian, gay, bisexual, transgender, queer, and HIV-affected hate violence in 2014: 2015 release edition.* New York: National Coalition of Anti-Violence Programs. Retrieved from www.avp.org/storage/documents/Reports/2014_HV_Report-Final.pdf

American Psychiatric Association. (1952). *Diagnostic and statistical manual of mental disorders* (DSM-I). Washington, D.C.: Author.

American Psychiatric Association. (1968). *Diagnostic and statistical manual of mental disorders* (2nd edition) (DSM-II). Washington, D.C.: Author.

American Psychiatric Association. (1980). *Diagnostic and statistical manual of mental disorders* (3rd edition-revised) (DSM-III-R). Washington, D.C.: Author.

American Psychiatric Association. (2000). *Diagnostic and statistical manual of mental disorders* (4th edition), *text revision* (DSM-IV-TR). Washington, D.C.: Author.

American Psychiatric Association. (2013). *Diagnostic and statistical manual of mental disorders* (5th edition) (DSM-5). Washington, DC: Author.

Associated Press. (2016, January 24). IOC rules transgender athletes can take part in Olympics without surgery. *The Guardian.* Retrieved from https://www.theguardian.com/sport/2016/jan/25/ioc-rules-transgender-athletes-can-take-part-in-olympics-without-surgery

Balbierz, P. (2014, January 29). Hijras: The battle for equality. *World Policy Blog.* Retrieved from www.worldpolicy.org/blog/2014/01/29/hijras-battle-equality

Beemyn, G. (2014). Transgender history in the United States. In L. Erickson-Schroth (Ed.) *Trans bodies, trans selves: A resource for the transgender community* (pp. 1–49). Oxford, UK: Oxford University Press.

Belluck, P. (2016, July). W.H.O. weighs dropping transgender identity from list of mental disorders. *The New York Times.* Retrieved from www.nytimes.com/2016/07/27/health/who-transgender-medical-disorder.html

Bilbrey, M. L. (2015). Transgender identity and media in historical perspective. *Honors Theses.* Retrieved from http://opensiuc.lib.siu.edu/cgi/viewcontent.cgi?article=1393&context=uhp_theses

Cauldwell, D.O. (2006). Psychopathia transexualis. In S. Stryker & S. Whittle (Eds.). *The Transgender Studies Reader* (40–44). London, UK: Routledge.

Clarke-Jervoise, S. & Smith, K. (2014–2016). *Boy Meets Girl* [Television Series]. London, England: BBC Two.

Cox, E. (2016, July 6). Boy Meets Girl and beyond: meet the transgender actors breaking new ground on British TV. *RadioTimes.* Retrieved from www.radiotimes.com/news/2016-07-06/boy-meets-girl-and-beyond-meet-the-transgender-actors-breaking-new-ground-on-british-tv

Csaky, Z. (2014, September 17). The east-west divide on LGBT rights in Europe. *Freedom House.* Retrieved from https://eeas.europa.eu/headquarters/headquarters-homepage/2810_en

Department of Health and Human Services, Office of the Secretary. (2016, May 18). Nondiscrimination in health programs and activities; Final rule. *Federal Register, 81(96)*, 31376–31473.

Drescher, J. (2016, August 15). Viewpoints: Gender diagnoses and ICD-11. *Psychiatric News.* Retrieved from http://psychnews.psychiatryonline.org/doi/full/10.1176/appi.pn.2016.8a15

Elders, M. J., Brown, G. R., Coleman, E., Kolditz, T. A., & Steinman, A. M. (2014). Medical aspects of transgender military service. *Armed Forces & Society, 41*(2), 1–22.

Emory, L. E., Williams, D. H., Cole, C. M., Amparo, E. G., & Meyer, W. J. (1991). Anatomic variation of the corpus callosum in persons with gender dysphoria. *Archives of Sexual Behavior, 20*(4), 409–417.

EU Spokesperson. (2016, May 12). Statement by the spokesperson on LGBTI rights in the United States. *European Union External Action*. Retrieved from https://eeas.europa.eu/headquarters/headquarters-homepage/2810_en

Freeman, G. (Producer). (1956–2016). *Eurovision Song Contest* [Television Series]. Le Grand-Saconnex, Switzerland: European Broadcasting Union & Sveriges Television.

Gansler, L. L. (2005). *The mysterious Private Thompson: The double life of Sarah Emma Edmonds, Civil War soldier.* New York, NY: Free Press.

Gates, G. J. & Herman, J. (2014). *Transgender military service in the United States.* Los Angeles, CA: Williams Institute, UCLA School of Law.

Gloucester County School Board v. G. G.. (n.d.). *Oyez*. Retrieved February 25, 2017, from https://www.oyez.org/cases/2016/16-273

Harrison-Quintana, J., & Herman, J. L. (2013). Still serving in silence: Transgender service members and veterans in the National Transgender Discrimination Survey. *LGBTQ Policy Journal, 3*(1), 1–13.

Harrod, H. (2016, February 28). The tragic true story behind *The Danish Girl*. *The Telegraph*. Retrieved from www.telegraph.co.uk/films/2016/04/14/the-tragic-true-story-behind-the-danish-girl/

Hitchcock, A. (Producer & Director). (1960). *Psycho* [Motion Picture]. United States: Paramount Pictures.

Hoffman, J. (2016, June 30). Estimate of U.S. transgender population doubles to 1.4 million adults. *New York Times*. Retrieved from www.nytimes.com/2016/07/01/health/transgender-population.html?ref=topics

James, S. E., Herman, J. L., Rankin, S., Keisling, M., Mottet, L., & Anafi, M. (2016). *The report of the 2015 U.S. transgender survey*. Washington, DC: National Center for Transgender Equality. Retrieved from www.transequality.org/sites/default/files/docs/usts/USTS%20Full%20Report%20-%20FINAL%201.6.17.pdf

Karasic, D. H. (2016). Protecting transgender rights promotes transgender health. *LGBT Health, 3*(4), 245-247.

Keck, T. M. (2009). Beyond backlash: Assessing the impact of judicial decisions on LGBT rights. *Law and Society Review, 43(1)*, 151-186.

Kidd, B. & Donnelly, P. (2000). Human rights in sports. *International Review for the Sociology of Sport, 35*(2), 131–148.

Klum, H. (Producer). (2006-2016). *Germany's Next Topmodel* [Television Series]. München, Germany: Tresor TV Produktions.

Kohan, J., Friedman, L., Hess, S., & Herrmann, T. (Producers). (2013–2016). *Orange is the New Black* [Television Series]. Los Gatos, CA: Netflix.

Luders, E., Sánchez, F. J., Tosun, D., Shattuck, D. W., Gaser, C., Vilain, E., & Toga, A. W. (2012). Increased cortical thickness in male-to-female transsexualism. *Journal of Behavioral and Brain Science, 2*(3), 357–362.

McCormick, J. P. (2015, May 16). Conchita Wurst: Some people think I'm a trans woman. *Pink News*. Retrieved from www.pinknews.co.uk/2015/05/16/conchita-wurst-some-people-get-me-confused-for-a-trans-woman/

Michaelson, J. (2015, February 23). America's deadly trans backlash. *The Daily Beast*. Retrieved from www.thedailybeast.com/articles/2015/02/23/the-hunting-of-trans-americans.html

Milliken, A. (2014, June 25). NYC Pride resolves issue over bisexual exclusion. *Pink News*. Retrieved from www.pinknews.co.uk/2014/06/25/nyc-pride-resolves-issue-over-bisexual-exclusion/

Money, J., Hampson, J. G., & Hampson, J. L. (1957). Imprinting and the establishment of gender role. *Archives of Neurology and Psychiatry*, 77(3), 333–336.

Mottet, L., & Tanis, J. (2008). *Opening the door to the inclusion of transgender people: The nine keys to making lesbian gay, bisexual and transgender organizations fully transgender-inclusive*. New York, NY: National Gay and Lesbian Task Force Policy Institute and the National Center for Transgender Equality.

NativeOUT Two Spirit Resource Center. (n.d.). Two spirit 101. In *Two Spirit Resource Center*. Retrieved from http://nativeout.com/twospirit-rc/two-spirit-101/

Outsports. (2016, July 11). A record 56 out LGBT athletes compete in Rio Olympics. *SB Nation*. Retrieved from www.outsports.com/2016/7/11/12133594/rio-olympics-teams-2016-gay-lgbt-athletes-record

Padawer, R. (2016, June 28). The humiliating practice of sex-testing female athletes. *The New York Times*. Retrieved from www.nytimes.com/2016/07/03/magazine/the-humiliating-practice-of-sex-testing-female-athletes.html

Pelleschi, A. (2016). *Transgender rights and issues*. Minneapolis, MN: Abdo Publishing.

Pink News. (2009, February 13). Transsexual win's battle to serve in Spain's armed forces. *Pink News*. Retrieved from www.pinknews.co.uk/2009/02/13/transsexual-wins-battle-to-serve-in-spains-armed-forces/

Pullin, Z. (2014, May-June). Two spirit: The story of a movement unfolds. *Native Peoples*. Retrieved from www.nativepeoples.com/Native-Peoples/May-June-2014/Two-Spirit-The-Story-of-a-Movement-Unfolds/

Reed, B., Rhodes, S., Schofield, P., & Wylie, K. (2009). *Gender variance in the UK: Prevalence, incidence, growth, and geographic distribution*. Surrey, UK: Gender Identity Research and Education Society. Retrieved from https://www.gires.org.uk/assets/Medpro-Assets/GenderVarianceUK-report.pdf

Reed, G. M., Drescher, J., Krueger, R. B., Atalla, E., Cochran, S. D., First, M. B., Cohen-Kettenis, P. T., Arango-de Montis, I., Parish, S. J., Cottler, S., Briken, P., Saxena, S. (2016). Disorders related to sexuality and gender identity in the ICD-11: revising the ICD-10 classification based on current scientific evidence, best clinical practices, and human rights considerations. *World Psychiatry*, *15*(3), 205–221.

Robles, R., Fresán, A., Vega-Ramírez, H., Cruz-Islas, J., Rodríguez-Pérez, V., Domínguez-Martínez, T. & Reed, G.M. (2016). Removing transgender identity from the classification of mental disorders: a Mexican field study for ICD-11. *Lancet Psychiatry*, *3*, 850–859.

Rudacille, D. (2005). *The Riddle of Gender*. New York, NY: Pantheon Books.

Sanchez, R. (2016, May 14). Feds' transgender guidance provokes fierce backlash. *CNN*. Retrieved from www.cnn.com/2016/05/14/politics/transgender-bathrooms-backlash/

Schwartz, Y. (2016, August 8). What the U.S. is learning from how Israel treats transgender soldiers. *Time*. Retrieved from http://time.com/4421400/transgender-u-s-military-israeli-army-idf/

Shalal, A. (2016, August 4). Germany high court rejects 'intersex' as third gender category. *Reuters*. Retrieved from www.reuters.com/article/us-germany-gender-idUSKCN10F2FB

Sharp, J., Kolodner, E., & Vachon, C. (Producers) & Peirce, K. (Director). (1999). *Boys Don't Cry* [Motion Picture]. United States: Fox Searchlight Pictures.

Sinisi, J.V. (2012). Gender non-conformity as a foundation for sex discrimination: Why Title IX may be an appropriate remedy for the NCAA transgender student-athletes. *Jeffrey S. Moorad Sports Law Journal, 19*(1), 343–369.

Stoller, R. (2006). Selection from biological substrates of sexual behavior. In S. Stryker & S. Whittle (Eds.). *The Transgender Studies Reader* (pp. 53–57). London, UK: Routledge.

Stryker, S. (2004). Transgender activism. In *glbtq Encyclopedia*. Retrieved from www.glbtqarchive.com/ssh/transgender_activism_S.pdf

Transgender Europe. (2016). *Trans Rights Europe Map & Index 2016*. Berlin, Germany: Transgender Europe. Retrieved from http://tgeu.org/trans-rights_europe_map_2016/

United States Department of Defense. (2016). *Transgender service in the U.S. military: An implementation handbook*. Retrieved from www.defense.gov/Portals/1/features/2016/0616_policy/DoDTGHandbook_093016.pdf?ver=2016-09-30-160933-837

Utt, K., Saxon, E., & Bozman, R. (Producers) & Demme, J., (Director). (1991). *The Silence of the Lambs* [Motion Picture]. United States: Orion.

von Krafft-Ebing, R. (1894/2012). *Pyschopathia sexualis, with especial reference to contrary sexual instinct: A medico-legal study.* London, UK: Forgotten Books.

White, M. (2012, April 26). End of gender: "Transsexual killer" strikes again. *Bitch media*. Retrieved from https://bitchmedia.org/post/end-of-gender-transsexual-killer-strikes-again-sevigny-transphobia

Witten, T.M. (2007). *Gender identity and the military - transgender, transsexual, and intersex identified individuals in the U.S. Armed Forces.* Santa Barbara, CA: Michael D. Palm Center, University of California, Santa Barbara. Retrieved from www.palmcenter.org/wp-content/uploads/2007/05/TransMilitary2007.pdf

World Health Organization. (1992). *International statistical classification of diseases and related health problems, 10th revision* (ICD-10). Geneva: WHO. Retrieved from www.who.int/classifications/icd/en/bluebook.pdf

World Professional Association for Transgender Health. (2011). *Standards of care for the health of transsexual, transgender, and gender nonconforming people, 7th edition*. Retrieved from https://s3.amazonaws.com/amo_hub_content/Association140/files/Standards%20of%20Care%20V7%20-%202011%20WPATH%20(2)(1).pdf

Zaimov, S. (2016, May 16). Target backlash over transgender bathroom policy hits 'boiling point,' business insiders say. *Christian Post*. Retrieved from www.christianpost.com/news/target-boycott-ransgender-bathroom-policy-hits-boiling-point-business-insider-says-163979/

Zucker, K. J., & Lawrence, A. A. (2009). Epidemiology of Gender Identity Disorder: Recommendations for the Standards of Care of the World Professional Association for Transgender Health. *International Journal of Transgenderism, 11*(1), 8–18.

3 The Intersectionality of Minority Identities and Health

John R. Blosnich, PhD, MPH

The views expressed in this material are those of the authors and do not reflect the official policy or position of the Department of Veterans Affairs or the U.S. Government.

In perhaps one of the most eloquent statements conveying the concept of intersectionality, author Audre Lorde wrote, "there is no such thing as a single-issue struggle, because we do not live single-issue lives" (Lorde, 1984). Intersectionality represents the idea that individuals' identities throughout the lifespan are shaped by gender identity, and race, and ethnicity, and socio-economic status, and sexual orientation, and being differently abled, and numerous other qualities (Collins, 2015). The excessive use of "and" in the previous sentence is intentional; simply put, intersectionality is about the "and." Applying an intersectionality approach to understanding health and health disparities is recognizing that a person may be lesbian *and* transgender *and* Latina *and* living with PTSD *and* residing in an economically depressed area. An intersectionality approach challenges providers and researchers to view health and its determinants as simultaneous and reciprocal interactions of multiple personal and social identities an individual has across the lifespan.

Another important principle of an intersectional approach is that identities should not be organized as a hierarchy. To suggest that one identity is more or less important resurrects the counterproductive categorization that an intersectional approach aims to avoid. Rather, identities should be approached as dynamic, interactive, with salience varying by situation and experience. In explaining intersectionality in terms of race and gender, Kimberle Crenshaw (1989) wrote:

> Black women sometimes experience discrimination in ways similar to white women's experiences; sometimes they share very similar experiences with Black men. Yet often they experience double-discrimination – the combined effects of practices, which discriminate on the basis of race, and on the basis of sex. And sometimes, they experience discrimination as Black women – not the sum of race and sex discrimination, but as Black women.
>
> (p.149)

Thus, we need to better understand the breadth of experiences that can act as determinants of health (such as discrimination). Assigning importance solely to one identity obscures unique factors that may only be revealed through a compound lens of multiple identities.

Minority Stress

Identities can become a source of stress due to societal stigma that attributes negative stereotypes and assumptions to specific identities. For example, gender is perhaps the most basic form of an identity because it often is attributed to individuals at birth (or even before birth through sonograms) and based on biological primary sex characteristics. Typically, it is anticipated that sex assigned at birth and gender will be concordant, that is, the person will be cisgender. Historically, many societies have viewed sex/gender as exclusively either male/masculine or female/feminine, and anyone not fitting into that socially constructed cisgender binary is viewed negatively as "other" and has their existence challenged or policed into compliance. While gender policing can be very clearly exemplified by the discrimination and harassment faced by transgender individuals, it also can affect non-transgender people (e.g., a boy who takes ballet classes being bullied by his peers for being gay or feminine because of the stereotype that ballet is "for girls").

The active (e.g., harassment, discrimination) and passive (e.g., exclusion of transgender identities) aggressions of gender policing are examples of *minority stress*, which refers to the distress individuals experience as a consequence of having a minority identity that is socially devalued and persecuted. Informed by seminal work on stigma by Erving Goffman in the 1960s (Goffman, 1963), Virginia Brooks (1981) was perhaps the first person to publish a discussion on the implications of minority stress and sexual orientation in her book focused on the experience of lesbian-identified women. Ilan Meyer moved this work forward through empirical investigation and developing a conceptual model to outline constructs involved in the processes of minority stress (Meyer, 2003).

While the complexities of the minority stress model are beyond the scope of this chapter [see Meyer (2003) for a detailed outline of the conceptual model of minority stress], the principal characteristics of minority stress that set it apart from typical stress are that it is unique, chronic, and socially-based (Meyer, 2003). Minority stress is unique in that it is additive to the typical stressors experienced by the general population; chronic in that it is rooted in perpetual sociocultural beliefs and practices that work to disadvantage minority identities; and socially-based in that the stress results from constructs and interactions that are beyond the individual. With an understanding of the concept of minority stress, it becomes clearer how intersectionality may moderate the level of distress a person may experience. For example, an African American, transgender woman may experience increased stress stemming from a complex maelstrom of racism *and* sexism *and* transphobia.

On a daily basis, she may not only face overt or covert racism but also endure sexist comments from men about her body, and dismissive looks from other women. To highlight one form of oppression as more important than another is to overlook the cumulative toll they all have on her health.

Stigma and Minority Stress

Societal stigma is an important component involved in minority stress processes and is likely a catalyst for minority stress. Hatzenbuehler and colleagues (2013) posit that the stigma that gives rise to minority stress is a major overlooked cause of health disparities. This framing to emphasize stigma as constituent of minority stress both helps to clarify minority stress processes and raises important implications for intervention. First, it expands the scope of the problem from the individual level of the person's psychology and re-emphasizes the gravity of the socially-based characteristic of minority stress. This shift in scope is paramount, because although psychotherapy and other individual-level treatments for distress are vital to intervening on the effects of minority stress, so too should science take a public health approach of *preventing* minority stress, which means combatting stigma. This focus on battling stigma takes the unique angle of also expanding the focus of interventions beyond the individual level. For example, a more comprehensive goal for promoting transgender health includes *both* individual level interventions (e.g., psychotherapy and pharmacotherapy to manage minority stress) *and* larger-scale activities to dismantle the transphobic social environmental factors that cause minority stress (e.g., implementing training and policies to assure equal and respectful service provision to transgender individuals).

This view of combatting stigma as a public health problem is relatively new to empirical research. However, there have been studies that show how sexual orientation-related stigma (e.g., anti-gay laws and policies, discrimination) is associated with increased prevalence of mental health problems among gay, lesbian, and bisexual individuals (Bostwick, Boyd, Hughes, West, & McCabe, 2014; Hatzenbuehler, Keyes, & Hasin, 2009; Hatzenbuehler, McLaughlin, Keyes, & Hasin, 2010; Lee, Gamarel, Bryant, Zaller, & Operario, 2016). One of the first studies to apply this methodology to transgender health found that transgender veterans who lived in states in the United States (U.S.) that had laws to protect transgender individuals from employment discrimination had lower odds of mood disorder diagnoses and lower odds of suicidal ideation or attempt than their transgender veteran peers who lived in states without employment discrimination protection (Blosnich et al., 2016). These examples elucidate the importance of context to understand health disparities, which in turn can inform treatment and prevention efforts.

Health Disparities among Transgender Populations

The increased burden of minority stress among transgender populations is thought to be a major driver of the numerous health disparities faced by this population. The literature on transgender populations can be understood as research focused on health risk behaviors versus health conditions. Due to the relatively new focus on transgender health in research and the limited data sources that include information about transgender status, a preponderance of literature has focused on disparities in health risk behaviors. Apart from studies about HIV, the literature is less developed in reporting about health conditions among transgender individuals for several reasons, including lack of self-reported data and the inability to examine electronic health record (EHR) data because transgender status is not included in most EHR systems.

Health Risk Disparities—Suicide

Perhaps the clearest areas of health risk disparities for transgender individuals are suicidal ideation and suicide attempt. There is a concordance of evidence from both self-report survey data and EHR data that transgender individuals have a starkly higher prevalence of lifetime suicidal ideation and suicide attempt than general population estimates. For example, several studies of convenience-based samples of transgender people have noted self-reported lifetime prevalence of suicidal ideation ranging between 37% to 65% (Kenagy, 2005; Lehavot, Simpson, & Shipherd, 2016; Mathy, 2003; McDuffie & Brown, 2010; Xavier, Honnold, & Bradford, 2007). As a point of comparison, lifetime suicidal ideation among the general U.S. adult population is estimated at 8.4% (Baca-Garcia et al., 2010) and approximately 9% in a large cross-national study of 60 countries (Nock et al., 2008). Studies of self-reported lifetime suicide attempt prevalence among transgender samples also noted starkly high estimates, ranging from 18% to 41% (Clements-Nolle, Marx, & Katz, 2006; Haas, Rodgers, & Herman, 2014; Lytle, Blosnich, & Kamen, 2016; Maguen & Shipherd, 2010; McDuffie & Brown, 2010; Xavier et al., 2007), while the estimated lifetime prevalence of suicide attempt among the general U.S. adult population is about 2.4% (Baca-Garcia et al., 2010) and approximately 2.7% worldwide (Nock et al., 2008). A study of EHR data from the Veterans Health Administration (VHA), found that transgender veterans utilizing VHA care (defined as veterans ever having a diagnosis of gender identity disorder), had a rate of serious suicidal ideation and suicide attempt that was approximately 20 times higher than the general population of veterans utilizing VHA care (Blosnich et al., 2013).

EHR data studies from European countries suggest that suicide mortality is elevated among specific subsamples of transgender populations, including Dutch transgender women receiving cross-sex hormone therapy (Asscheman, Giltay, Megens, van Trotsenburg, & Gooren, 2011; Asscheman, Gooren, & Eklund, 1989; Van Kesteren, Asscheman, Megens, & Gooren, 1997) and Swedish individuals who had undergone gender confirming surgery (Dhejne et al., 2011). In the U.S., VHA data on transgender veterans noted not only a high rate of suicide mortality, but also a greater burden of years of potential life lost because transgender veterans who died by suicide were, on average, younger than the general metrics of VHA veterans who died by suicide (Blosnich, Brown, Wojcio, Jones, & Bossarte, 2014).

Other Health Disparities

Transgender individuals also experience high rates of health risks in the forms of discrimination, rejection, and interpersonal violence. For example, in the U.S. Transgender Survey (USTS) of over 27,000 transgender and gender non-conforming individuals, approximately 1 in 10 had lost a job because of their gender identity, and the unemployment rate for the sample was 3 times higher than the unemployment rate for the general U.S. population at the time of the survey (James et al., 2016). In addition to discrimination, transgender individuals also face family rejection. In the USTS, 50% of the sample reported experiencing rejection by their families, and evidence from qualitative research includes narratives of being cast out of the home and physical, verbal, and emotional abuse from parents (Grossman & D'augelli, 2006; James et al., 2016; Koken, Bimbi, & Parsons, 2009). Transgender individuals also experience considerable violence from persons outside their families. One study of transgender people found nearly universal exposure to trauma, with 98% reporting at least one potentially traumatic event and 42% saying the trauma was related to transgender bias (Shipherd, Maguen, Skidmore & Abramovitz, 2011). In addition, there are very high rates of sexual assault (Stotzer, 2009). For instance, in one of the largest comparative studies of a U.S. transgender population, Brown and Jones (2016) examined health disparities between transgender and non-transgender veterans, finding that transgender veterans had over 2.5 times the odds of reporting military sexual trauma (MST) compared to non-transgender veterans. Moreover, in a study specifically comparing black transgender veterans and white transgender veterans, Brown and Jones (2014) noted several differences, such as greater prevalence of HIV, congestive heart failure, hypertension, and end-stage renal disease among Black transgender veterans.

Other health risks documented among samples of transgender individuals include commercial sex work and survival sex (Herbst et al., 2008; Walls & Bell, 2011), homelessness (James et al., 2016), incarceration (Brown & McDuffie, 2009; Clements-Nolle, Marx, Guzman, & Katz, 2001), cigarette smoking (Conron, Scott, Stowell, & Landers, 2012), alcohol abuse (Coulter et al., 2015), and barriers to accessing health care (Sanchez, Sanchez, & Danoff, 2009; Sevelius, Patouhas, Keatley, & Johnson, 2014; Shipherd, Green, & Abramovitz, 2010; Shipherd, Mizock, Maguen, & Green, 2012). In addition, evidence clearly suggests that transgender individuals—particularly transgender women—are overrepresented among people living with HIV in the U.S. (Baral et al., 2013). Research has begun to uncover other potential disparities transgender populations may face, including hepatitis C infection (Porter, Lusk, & Katz, 2014) and co-infection of other sexually transmitted diseases with HIV (Chu et al., 2012).

Limitations of Current Research

The current literature portrays a landscape in which transgender individuals bear large burdens of disparities both in terms of health risks and health conditions. There are, however, at least two major limitations in summarizing the current literature and synthesizing results in order to appraise how this information may bear on providing mental health care to transgender clients. First, the sampling designs across studies—from reliance on convenience-based samples to EHR data—inhibit the generalizability of the results. For example, several studies using a census sample of transgender veterans receiving VHA care have created new opportunities for learning about transgender health (Blosnich et al., 2013; Brown & Jones, 2016; Kauth et al., 2014), however these studies are limited to veterans and, more specifically, to U.S. veterans who receive VHA care for gender identity concerns. Second, many of the current studies of transgender samples do not include a non-transgender comparison sample, so adequately gauging the extent of disparity is difficult and must often be compared to general population estimates.

Transgender health research stands to increase in volume and quality as gender identity items are incorporated into federal, national, and international health surveys, increasing the ability to have direct comparison groups and data that are more generalizable to the general population metrics (The GenIUSS Group, 2014).

Thinking about the Intersections of Health Disparities

Where intersectionality provides a framework for understanding the numerous social identities individuals have and the unique and interactive effects these identities have on health, *syndemic theory* outlines how health risks, conditions, and disparities interact; a confluence of epidemics. Specifically, medical anthropologist Merrill Singer defines a syndemic as "a set of enmeshed and mutually enhancing health problems that, working together in a context of noxious social and physical conditions, can significantly affect the overall disease burden and health status of a population" (Singer, 2009, p. xiv). The important characteristic of a syndemic approach is that any one condition is made worse by its interaction with other conditions, and that treating or reducing any one condition is predicated on addressing those interactions.

While most providers may be familiar with the concept of co-morbidity (the co-occurrence of health conditions), syndemic theory expands the view of co-morbidity beyond individually-diagnosed health conditions. Although health conditions are parts of a syndemic approach, syndemic theory also includes the social processes that contribute to or worsen health conditions. A syndemic approach helps to map negative feedback loops and allows for "unpacking" the multiple factors that contribute to, are results of, or are both contributors to and results of conditions. Singer's classic example of syndemic theory was his examination of the intertwined health problems of substance abuse, violence, and AIDS (SAVA) among Puerto Rican adolescent and adult individuals living in an urban area (Singer & Hispanic Health Council, 2000). Not only did individuals experience the negative consequences of illicit drug use, their gang involvement resulted in being both victims and perpetrators of violence, all of which created an environment that elevated the risk of HIV infection.

Singer's example also illustrates how other elements of the syndemic can undercut the effectiveness of an intervention for one particular problem. For example, an HIV education or treatment adherence program may encounter significant challenges in recruitment, attendance, or retention because the risk of gang violence precludes where, when, and how individuals travel. The intended population may also miss their appointments because of their illicit drug use. The syndemic combination of all these elements must be addressed for effective intervention to occur.

Figure 3.1 portrays an example of thinking about the syndemic production of suicidal ideation in a client named Susan. Susan recently conveyed to her mental health provider that she has been having serious thoughts of taking her own life. Initially, her provider believed this stemmed from Susan's alcohol use. She often commented how drinking helps her to forget about the world, but she always reaches a point where "it doesn't work anymore, and that makes me feel even worse" (C). At times, she resorted to harder substances to deal with her depression, only to feel worse about herself when the high wore off (F). On numerous occasions she has admitted, "when I booze I use, when I use I booze" regarding her use of illicit drugs (B). Susan also has recurring housing instability. She is depressed when her friends tell her that she can no longer stay with them because of her drug use (A, D, E). Her depression keeps her from completing paperwork for a local housing program (D), reinforced by her hopelessness to be drug-free, which is a requirement of the housing program (A). When she cannot find shelter, she resorts to spaces where drug and alcohol use are rampant (A, E).

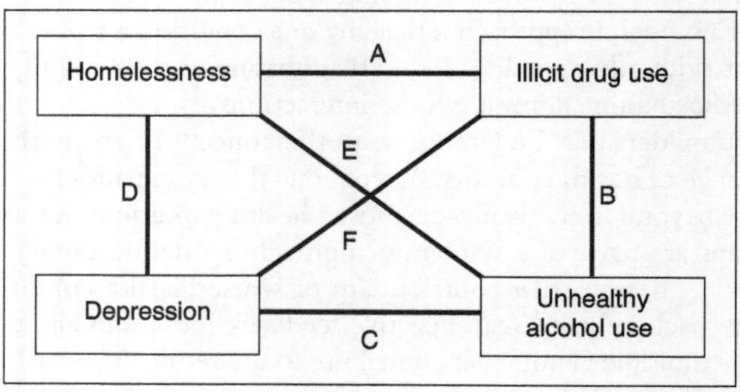

Figure 3.1 Syndemic example

In Susan's case, it is not simply depression *or* alcohol abuse *or* illicit drug use *or* homelessness that solely leads to her suicidal ideation. Again, as with an intersectionality approach, this is an example of changing the "or" to "and" to better understand the individual's experience and help the individual set realistic goals and mutually decide where and how to intervene to meet those goals. The landscape of health is complex and dynamic, which challenges providers to develop complex and dynamic strategies for treatment.

Clinical Case Examples

This section briefly illustrates the complexities of intersecting identities and how these different identities are important to the individual. Following each case, there are questions you may ask yourself while formulating your treatment plan with each client.

1. Yelena is a 62-year-old transgender woman seeking treatment for her depression, which she has managed periodically since she was diagnosed as an adolescent. This is her third visit with you, having been referred to your practice by a local community service organization. Her first visit was about 6 weeks ago, and since then you have learned a lot about Yelena, but she is guarded and you are still forming a rapport with her. Yelena waited to transition until she was 48, after her beloved but very traditional Latina grandmother had passed away. However, since her transition, many members of her biological family have refused to communicate with her, saying that her transition was something not supported by their Latino culture and Catholic faith. She learned that her uncle had passed away recently, and she was saddened by the fact that the family had not wanted her to come to the funeral, reigniting her depression about issues with her family.

   In addition to the recurrence of her familial conflict, Yelena works as a server at a local restaurant, a place at which she has worked for almost 5 years. While the management and her co-workers are supportive to her, sometimes the patrons are not. Last week, she caught a group of young women, whom she was serving, pointing and laughing at her when they thought she could not see them. When she brought their food, one woman commented on how her large hands could handle so many plates while the other women hid their laughter. They didn't leave her a tip, but left a tube of old lipstick with a hastily scratched note on the receipt that read, "Real women wear makeup." Yelena said she typically ignores this type of harassment, citing that it happens all the time, but that she must have been feeling particularly bad because of the news of her uncle's passing.

   Finally, she is becoming increasingly worried about the landlord of her new apartment. When she first moved in, he was more than happy to help her move some of her belongings, but she got the impression he was trying to flirt with her. Not wanting to anger him, or risk being kicked out of the apartment, she tried to laugh off his excessive compliments and ignored his frequent touching of her arm. Lately, however, his advances have become more overt, and a few days ago he mentioned how he had always been attracted to Latina women because they are "so exotic," and that if she wanted to save on rent, Yelena could always pay him "in other ways." While she isn't sure what precisely brought on her latest bout of depression, she feels like the weight of the world is becoming too much for her to handle.

As her treating provider, how does Yelena see herself? What additional information do you need to ask for that would help in formulating a treatment plan? What identities are important to her? In what ways are her identities in conflict? Is Yelena at physical risk? How can you engage and help Yelena? How can you validate the real discrimination she has experienced while offering hope for the future by identifying ways to increase safety? How will you determine what is most important to Yelena as a place to begin work?

2. Levi is a 26-year-old U.S. Army veteran who has been hospitalized for a suspected suicide attempt, though he contends he simply misread the instructions on painkillers he was taking for a back injury. He was honorably discharged after serving two tours in Iraq and one tour in Afghanistan, where he was injured by an improvised explosive device, which also killed two of his friends in his unit. However, during his time in the Army, he was known as and lived as Darlene, as his sex assigned at birth was female. He started his transition after leaving the Army for fear of being discharged and losing his benefits if anyone found out he identified as a transgender man. Levi receives care from you at the local VHA medical center for depression and for posttraumatic stress disorder (PTSD) attributed to events that occurred serving in combat. He also carries a diagnosis of gender dysphoria that is currently well-controlled through prior surgeries and hormone treatment. He has been your client for just over a year now, and you believe you have a very good, open rapport with him. However, unbeknownst to you, he still is not able to bring himself to disclose that he has PTSD symptoms related to repeated sexual harassment and a sexual assault that occurred during his military service.

Since he began his transition, he has distanced himself from his mother, Raynelle, who cried when she found out he had a double mastectomy. She refuses to call him Levi or use male pronouns when referring to him. Raynelle, recognizing some symptoms of PTSD, appealed to Levi to begin re-attending their African Methodist Episcopal church, saying that meditation and prayer are what he needs. When Raynelle found out about the mastectomy, she lamented that "Darlene" was not going to be able to give her grandchildren, and that she was running out of excuses to tell people about why he doesn't come home anymore. He now sends his mother's calls to voicemail and has not spoken with her in nearly 6 months.

Levi resumed his work on heavy equipment maintenance, skills he learned while in the Army, and has worked for an oil and gas company for the past 2 years. None of his co-workers know he is a transgender man, and he is extremely fearful of any of them finding out. He is used to hearing racist remarks from some of the men on the crew. These men think they are joking with Levi, who is actually highly bothered by the remarks, but tries to laugh them off in order to avoid escalating the situations. He is the only African American person on his crew, and besides one other Latino mechanic, Levi is the only person of color in the entire shop. He doubts his management would support him if he filed a complaint.

Levi has always considered weight-training one of his best stress management tools, but lately he feels like it is a necessity in order to protect himself. He increased his gym visits to twice daily during the week and has also been thinking about increasing his testosterone on his own without telling his doctor. A friend who he corresponds with, who also is a transgender man, gave him some advice on how to get extra testosterone online. However, Levi's extreme training regimen is exacerbating the back injury he sustained from his time in the military, and when he cannot train or has to skip a day, he starts to worry that the results he has worked so hard for will erode.

As his treating provider, how does Levi see himself? What identities are important to him? In what ways are his identities in conflict? How can you engage with him to discuss previous traumas (i.e., military sexual assault) that he is reluctant to share? In what ways are his coping strategies helpful and in what ways are they putting his health at risk? What kind of social support does Levi have and how can it be increased? How might you engage and help Levi? How will you determine what is most important to Levi as a place to begin work?

Take-Home Points

- An intersectionality approach outlines a way of understanding health as a function of the many identities a person holds across the life course and the interaction between those identities and society.
- Minority stress, originating from stigma, likely gives rise to the many health risk and health condition disparities found in transgender populations.
- Syndemic theory offers a framework for critically thinking about how health problems are linked and, together, create worse health outcomes. This theory expands the focus of treatment from a single health problem to the ties that bind health problems together.

Recommended Reading

Cole, E. R. (2009). Intersectionality and research in psychology. *American Psychologist, 64*(3), 170–180.

Hatzenbuehler, M. L. (2009). How does sexual minority stigma "get under the skin"? A psychological mediation framework. *Psychological Bulletin, 135*(5), 707–730.

Singer, M., & Clair, S. (2003). Syndemics and public health: Reconceptualizing disease in bio-social context. *Medical Anthropology Quarterly, 17*(4), 423–441.

References

Asscheman, H., Giltay, E. J., Megens, J. A. J., van Trotsenburg, M. A. A., & Gooren, L. J. G. (2011). A long-term follow-up study of mortality in transsexuals receiving treatment with cross-sex hormones. *European Journal of Endocrinology, 164*(4), 635–642.

Asscheman, H., Gooren, L., & Eklund, P. (1989). Mortality and morbidity in transsexual patients with cross-gender hormone treatment. *Metabolism, 38*(9), 869–873.

Baca-Garcia, E., Perez-Rodriguez, M. M., Keyes, K. M., Oquendo, M. A., Hasin, D. S., Grant, B. F., & Blanco, C. (2010). Suicidal ideation and suicide attempts in the United States: 1991–1992 and 2001–2002. *Molecular Psychiatry, 15*(3), 250–259.

Baral, S. D., Poteat, T., Strömdahl, S., Wirtz, A. L., Guadamuz, T. E., & Beyrer, C. (2013). Worldwide burden of HIV in transgender women: a systematic review and meta-analysis. *The Lancet Infectious Diseases, 13*(3), 214–222.

Blosnich, J. R., Brown, G. R., Shipherd, P., Jillian C, Kauth, M., Piegari, R. I., & Bossarte, R. M. (2013). Prevalence of gender identity disorder and suicide risk among transgender veterans utilizing Veterans Health Administration care. *American Journal of Public Health, 103*(10), e27–e32.

Blosnich, J. R., Brown, G. R., Wojcio, S., Jones, K. T., & Bossarte, R. M. (2014). Mortality among veterans with transgender-related diagnoses in the Veterans Health Administration, FY2000–2009. *LGBT Health, 1*(4), 269–276.

Blosnich, J. R., Marsiglio, M. C., Gao, S., Gordon, A. J., Shipherd, J. C., Kauth, M., & Fine, M. J. (2016). Mental health of transgender veterans in US states with and without discrimination and hate crime legal protection. *American Journal of Public Health, 106*(3), 534–540.

Bostwick, W. B., Boyd, C. J., Hughes, T. L., West, B. T., & McCabe, S. E. (2014). Discrimination and mental health among lesbian, gay, and bisexual adults in the United States. *American Journal of Orthopsychiatry, 84*(1), 35.

Brooks, V. R. (1981). *Minority stress and lesbian women*. Lexington, MA: Lexington Books.

Brown, G. R., & Jones, K. T. (2014). Racial health disparities in a cohort of 5,135 transgender veterans. *Journal of Racial and Ethnic Health Disparities, 1*(4), 257–266.

Brown, G. R., & Jones, K. T. (2016). Mental health and medical health disparities in 5135 transgender veterans receiving healthcare in the Veterans Health Administration: A case-control study. *LGBT Health, 3*(2), 122–131.

Brown, G. R., & McDuffie, E. (2009). Health care policies addressing transgender inmates in prison systems in the United States. *Journal of Correctional Health Care.*

Chu, P. L., Santos, G. M., Vu, A., Nieves-Rivera, I., Colfax, G. N., Grinsdale, J., Huang, S., Philip, S., Scheer, S., & Aragon, T. (2012). *Impact of syndemics on people living with HIV in San Francisco*. Paper presented at the XIX International AIDS Conference, Washington, DC.

Clements-Nolle, K., Marx, R., Guzman, R., & Katz, M. (2001). HIV prevalence, risk behaviors, health care use, and mental health status of transgender persons: Implications for public health intervention. *American Journal of Public Health, 91*(6), 915.

Clements-Nolle, K., Marx, R., & Katz, M. (2006). Attempted suicide among transgender persons: The influence of gender-based discrimination and victimization. *Journal of Homosexuality, 51*(3), 53–69.

Collins, P. H. (2015). Intersectionality's definitional dilemmas. *Annual Review of Sociology, 41*, 1–20.

Conron, K. J., Scott, G., Stowell, G. S., & Landers, S. J. (2012). Transgender health in Massachusetts: Results from a household probability sample of adults. *American Journal of Public Health, 102*(1), 118–122.

Coulter, R. W., Blosnich, J. R., Bukowski, L. A., Herrick, A., Siconolfi, D. E., & Stall, R. D. (2015). Differences in alcohol use and alcohol-related problems between transgender-and nontransgender-identified young adults. *Drug and Alcohol Dependence, 154*, 251–259.

Crenshaw, K. (1989). Demarginalizing the intersection of race and sex: A black feminist critique of antidiscrimination doctrine, feminist theory and antiracist politics. *University of Chicago Legal Forum, 140*, 139–167. Retrieved from http://chicagounbound.uchicago.edu/cgi/viewcontent.cgi?article=1052&context=uclf

Dhejne, C., Lichtenstein, P., Boman, M., Johansson, A. L., Långström, N., & Landén, M. (2011). Long-term follow-up of transsexual persons undergoing sex reassignment surgery: Cohort study in Sweden. *PloS-ONE, 6*(2), e16885. Retrieved from http://journals.plos.org/plosone/article?id=10.1371/journal.pone.0016885

Goffman, E. (1963). *Stigma: Notes on the management of spoiled identity*. New York, NY: Simon & Schuster.

Grossman, A. H., & D'augelli, A. R. (2006). Transgender youth: Invisible and vulnerable. *Journal of Homosexuality, 51*(1), 111–128.

Haas, A. P., Rodgers, P. L., & Herman, J. L. (2014). *Suicide attempts among transgender and gender non-conforming adults: Findings of the National Transgender Discrimination Survey*. Los Angeles, CA: The Williams Institute. Retreived from https://williamsinstitute.law.ucla.edu/wp-content/uploads/AFSP-Williams-Suicide-Report-Final.pdf

Hatzenbuehler, M. L., Keyes, K. M., & Hasin, D. S. (2009). State-level policies and psychiatric morbidity in lesbian, gay, and bisexual populations. *American Journal of Public Health, 99*(12), 2275–2281.

Hatzenbuehler, M. L., McLaughlin, K. A., Keyes, K. M., & Hasin, D. S. (2010). The impact of institutional discrimination on psychiatric disorders in lesbian, gay, and bisexual populations: A prospective study. *American Journal of Public Health, 100*(3), 452–459.

Hatzenbuehler, M. L., Phelan, J. C., & Link, B. G. (2013). Stigma as a fundamental cause of population health inequalities. *American Journal of Public Health, 103*(5), 813–821.

Herbst, J. H., Jacobs, E. D., Finlayson, T. J., McKleroy, V. S., Neumann, M. S., Crepaz, N., & Team, H. A. P. R. S. (2008). Estimating HIV prevalence and risk behaviors of transgender persons in the United States: A systematic review. *AIDS and Behavior, 12*(1), 1–17.

James, S., Herman, J. L., Rankin, S., Keisling, M., Mottet, L. A., & Anafi, M. (2016). *The report of the 2015 U.S. Transgender Survey*. Washington, D.C.: National Center for Transgender Equality. Retrieved from www.transequality.org/sites/default/files/docs/usts/USTS%20Full%20Report%20-%20FINAL%201.6.17.pdf

Kauth, M. R., Shipherd, J. C., Lindsay, J., Blosnich, J. R., Brown, G. R., & Jones, K. T. (2014). Access to care for transgender veterans in the Veterans Health Administration: 2006–2013. *American Journal of Public Health, 104*(S4), S532–S534.

Kenagy, G. P. (2005). Transgender health: Findings from two needs assessment studies in Philadelphia. *Health & Social Work, 30*(1), 19–26.

Koken, J. A., Bimbi, D. S., & Parsons, J. T. (2009). Experiences of familial acceptance–rejection among transwomen of color. *Journal of Family Psychology, 23*(6), 853–860.

Lee, J. H., Gamarel, K. E., Bryant, K. J., Zaller, N. D., & Operario, D. (2016). Discrimination, mental health, and substance use disorders among sexual minority populations. *LGBT Health, 3*(4), 258–265.

Lehavot, K., Simpson, T. L., & Shipherd, J. C. (2016). Factors associated with suicidality among a national sample of transgender veterans. *Suicide and Life-Threatening Behavior, 46*(5), 507–524.

Lorde, A. (1984). *Sister outsider: Essays and speeches*. Berkeley, CA: Crossing Press.

Lytle, M. C., Blosnich, J. R., & Kamen, C. (2016). The association of multiple identities with self-directed violence and depression among transgender individuals. *Suicide and Life-Threatening Behavior, 46*(5), 535–544.

Maguen, S., & Shipherd, J. C. (2010). Suicide risk among transgender individuals. *Psychology & Sexuality, 1*(1), 34–43.

Mathy, R. M. (2003). Transgender identity and suicidality in a nonclinical sample: Sexual orientation, psychiatric history, and compulsive behaviors. *Journal of Psychology & Human Sexuality, 14*(4), 47–65.

McDuffie, E., & Brown, G. R. (2010). 70 US veterans with gender identity disturbances: A descriptive study. *International Journal of Transgenderism, 12*(1), 21–30.

Meyer, I. H. (2003). Prejudice, social stress, and mental health in lesbian, gay, and bisexual populations: Conceptual issues and research evidence. *Psychological Bulletin, 129*, 643–658.

Nock, M. K., Borges, G., Bromet, E. J., Alonso, J., Angermeyer, M., Beautrais, A., Bruffaerts, R., Chiu, W. T., De Girolamo, G., & Gluzman, S. (2008). Cross-national prevalence and risk factors for suicidal ideation, plans and attempts. *The British Journal of Psychiatry, 192*(2), 98–105.

Porter, J. C., Lusk, H. M., & Katz, A. R. (2014). Prevalence of HCV infection among clients in community-based health settings in Hawaii, 2002–2010: Assessing risk factors. *American Journal of Public Health, 104*(8), 1534–1539.

Sanchez, N. F., Sanchez, J. P., & Danoff, A. (2009). Health care utilization, barriers to care, and hormone usage among male-to-female transgender persons in New York City. *American Journal of Public Health, 99*(4), 713–719.

Sevelius, J. M., Patouhas, E., Keatley, J. G., & Johnson, M. O. (2014). Barriers and facilitators to engagement and retention in care among transgender women living with human immunodeficiency virus. *Annals of Behavioral Medicine, 47*(1), 5–16.

Shipherd, J. C., Green, K. E., & Abramovitz, S. (2010). Transgender clients: Identifying and minimizing barriers to mental health treatment. *Journal of Gay & Lesbian Mental Health, 14*(2), 94–108.

Shipherd, J. C., Maguen, S., Skidmore, W. C., & Abramovitz, S. M. (2011). Potentially traumatic events in a transgender sample: Frequency and associated symptoms. *Traumatology, 17*(2), 56–67.

Shipherd, J. C., Mizock, L., Maguen, S., & Green, K. E. (2012). Male-to-female transgender veterans and VA health care utilization. *International Journal of Sexual Health, 24*(1), 78–87.

Singer, M. (2009). *Introduction to syndemics: A critical systems approach to public and community health*. San Francisco, CA: Jossey-Bass.

Singer, M., & Hispanic Health Council. (2000). A dose of drugs, a touch of violence, a case of AIDS: Conceptualizing the SAVA syndemic. *Free Inquiry*, *28*(1), 13–23.

Stotzer, R. L. (2009). Violence against transgender people: A review of United States data. *Aggression and Violent Behavior*, *14*(3), 170–179.

The GenIUSS Group. (2014). *Best practices for asking questions to identify transgender and other gender minority respondents on population-based surveys*. Los Angeles, CA: The Williams Institute. Retrieved from https://williamsinstitute.law.ucla.edu/wp-content/uploads/geniuss-report-sep-2014.pdf

Van Kesteren, P. J., Asscheman, H., Megens, J. A., & Gooren, L. J. (1997). Mortality and morbidity in transsexual subjects treated with cross-sex hormones. *Clinical Endocrinology*, *47*(3), 337–343.

Walls, N. E., & Bell, S. (2011). Correlates of engaging in survival sex among homeless youth and young adults. *Journal of Sex Research*, *48*(5), 423–436.

Xavier, J., Honnold, J. A., & Bradford, J. (2007). *The health, health-related needs, and lifecourse experiences of transgender Virginians*. Richmond, VA: Virginia Commonwealth University.

4 Providing a Welcoming Clinic Environment

Bryan N. Cochran, PhD
Oakleigh M. Reed, BS
Hillary A. Gleason, MA

Mental health professionals, as focused as we are on immediately engaging the individual, can easily lose sight of what the experience might be like for a new client walking through the door. It is a useful exercise for us to consider the possible mindset of the client in this situation. What does this client think about mental health professionals or about what it means to be "in therapy"? What does the client think that therapists are trained to do? Does the client believe that a new therapist will be able to understand their struggles and truly see who they are as a person?

This perspective-taking is particularly important when working with transgender and gender non-conforming clients. The legacy of the mental health profession's treatment of transgender individuals includes pathologization, conflating gender identity with sexual orientation, serving as a gatekeeper to medically necessary services, and discouraging individuals from expressing their authentic identities. Transgender individuals are likely to be *correct* that mental health professionals learned nothing about transgender identity, health disparities of transgender people, or the World Professional Association of Transgender Health *Standards of Care* (WPATH SOC) while in graduate school (Austin & Craig, 2015). Due to these training deficits, transgender individuals, aware that they may very well be the first transgender client a provider has seen, often take on the role of educating providers on the history of discrimination and mistreatment of the transgender community. Considering this perspective affords insight as to why transgender individuals may be tentative or on guard when seeking out new providers.

In terms of historical context, the experiences of transgender individuals have largely been ignored in the field of mental health. One exception was the pioneering work of Magnus Hirschfeld (1923/1984), who is credited with having first differentiated between sexual identities (i.e., those who wish to have partners of the same sex) and what he considered "transsexualism" (i.e., those who wish to live as another sex) almost a century ago. Note, though, that the term "transsexualism" is now considered an out-of-date term due to it often being conflated with disorders of sexuality. Unfortunately, much of Hirschfeld's work was lost or suppressed by the Nazi regime, and gender identity was presented in the literature largely as pathological for many subsequent decades.

References to transgender identity in the intervening years occur almost exclusively in abnormal psychology volumes and texts. The prevailing belief for many years was that for transgender, non-binary, or gender non-conforming individuals early developmental traumas or parenting problems resulted in identity confusion, and therefore transgender identity was something to be cured, not celebrated.

Many American providers are surprised to find out how much their transgender clients know about the Diagnostic and Statistical Manual (DSM) of Mental Disorders, just as European providers discover their transgender clients are informed about the International Classification of Diseases (ICD). Our perspective is that it makes sense for clients to be well apprised of manuals that have historically pathologized them simply for being who they are. In Chapter 2, an excellent overview of the historical pathologization of transgender identities is provided for context; the legacy of mistreatment by the mental health establishment is clear.

The reminder that "those who cannot remember the past are condemned to repeat it" (Santayana, 1905, p. 82) is relevant here: Providers who lack an understanding of the historical mistreatment of transgender individuals by the mental health establishment may, either explicitly or implicitly, replicate this mistreatment through their interactions with clients. Providers should consider the way this history continues to impact treatment seeking when setting up an affirmative and inclusive mental health environment.

Mental Health Help-Seeking among Transgender Individuals

Recent data from the 2015 United States (U.S.) Transgender Survey indicated that 39% of transgender respondents had experienced serious psychological distress within a month prior to completing the survey (James et al., 2016). This is a striking statistic when compared with only 5% of the general U.S. population reporting similar distress (James et al., 2016). It is critical to recognize that the hardships that transgender individuals encounter in social, occupational, and educational settings (among many others), also permeate the very places that are meant to aid the distress associated with these experiences. This same report also found that 33% of respondents had at least one negative experience with a health care provider in the past year (e.g., verbal harassment, discrimination based on gender identity; James et al., 2016). Additionally, 23% of respondents reported that they avoided seeking mental health care due to the fear of being mistreated (James et al., 2016). Further, 40% of transgender individuals had attempted suicide in their lifetime, which is nine times the rate in the general U.S. population (4.6%; James et al., 2016). Thus, it is important for providers to recognize both historical context and the personal negative experiences transgender individuals have faced in order to create an environment for them to safely navigate their gender identity, pursue a healthy social and/or physical transition (if desired), and address general psychological distress.

In preparation for the writing of this chapter, we thought it would be useful to survey transgender individuals about their utilization of mental health services. In a brief online survey, we inquired about individuals' positive and negative experiences accessing mental health care, and we also asked what mental health professionals should do to provide better services for transgender clients. Although we did not formally analyze these data, we have included quotes from the 77 individuals who completed our survey throughout this chapter to emphasize key points. Note that because people self-selected into the survey, these results should not be construed as representative of *all* transgender individuals. Also, although the term transgender is used throughout this volume as an umbrella term for identities, we utilized individuals' self-descriptions here (e.g., transguy, non-binary) along with their quotes to most accurately represent the identities they reported in the survey. Of these individuals, 84.4% (n=65) were either currently in therapy or had been in the past. Over half (n=41, 53.3%) had met with a mental health provider because doing so was required for access to transition-related services, but a greater number (n=49, 63.6%) had sought treatment for some other reason unrelated to gender identity (there is overlap between these two groups). We have also integrated the information gleaned from this survey, the relevant literature, and our professional experiences into a series of action steps, listed in Table 4.1. These steps will aid providers in creating a welcoming environment for transgender clients.

Table 4.1 Action steps to creating a welcoming environment

Action step	*Description*	*Example(s)*
1. Take the client's perspective	• Imagine what it is like to seek mental health treatment as a person who identifies as transgender. • Consider your health care environment's unique climate regarding transgender sensitivity, historically and presently. Your workplace and broader community may have a specific reputation or set of norms that could affect gender minority individuals' sense of acceptance and safety. • Use person-first language to respect clients' identities. • Consider your record system and potential challenges with documentation and billing. Address these systems prior to meeting with client to assure that you can help them make informed choices.	• *Anticipate things that would feel welcoming or not: e.g., visual clinic environment, mannerisms, paperwork, and other factors that would otherwise not be noticed without this perspective taking.* • *Research your community and organization's policies regarding gender inclusivity and non-discrimination.* • *Notice the difference between "a transgender woman seeking treatment at our clinic named Patient B" and "Patient B is seeking treatment at our clinic; she identifies as a transgender woman."* • *Does the electronic medical record allow for both legal name and preferred name. Does preferred name get sent to billing thereby "outing" the client to insurance?*

Action step	*Description*	*Example(s)*
2. Ask about gender identity	• Ask explicitly about gender identity, transgender status, and gender pronouns with <u>*all*</u> clients. ○ Consider introducing yourself with your gender pronouns and then ask the client which pronouns they prefer (either verbally or on paperwork). This will clarify what gender pronouns are employed for clients who are not used to hearing this question, and it sets up the expectation that gender is a comfortable topic of conversation. • Pronouns (including non-binary options such as "they/their") can be displayed prominently in the health record to help other professionals to avoid misgendering clients. • Use the two-step system to inquire about sex assigned at birth and gender identity. Some transgender individuals identify solely with the labels of "man" or "woman;" moreover, requiring transgender individuals to identify as "transgender man" or "transgender woman" but not having cisgender individuals identify as "cisman" or "ciswoman" is *othering* to gender minorities. The two-step system allows individuals to identify with whichever gender labels they prefer, while simultaneously collecting information about transgender status. The questions and responses in the following column model the two-step system. ○ Asking about gender identity and transgender status can signal to a client that you are open and comfortable with discussing transgender-related issues.	• *Example: "My name is Hillary, and I use the pronouns 'she' and 'hers.' What pronouns do you go by?"* a. *Note: We avoid the language of "preferred pronouns" here because it insinuates that gender is just a desire, rather than an identity. Language is important!* • *Step 1: "What sex were you assigned at birth?"* ○ *While it is ideal for clients to self-identify by writing their assigned sex and gender identity on an open line, this is sometimes complicated by records that call for a close-ended response. In this case, you can have clients check all that apply from "Female," "Male," and "Intersex"* ○ *Note: It is important to have clients check all that apply here rather than just one, because individuals who are intersex are also assigned a sex at birth.* • *Step 2: "What is your gender identity?"* ○ *Again, it is ideal for clients to be able to write down their gender identity label. However, when closed responses are necessary, clients can check all that apply from "Woman," "Man," "Genderqueer," "Two-Spirit," "Other gender identity: ___________."*

(continued)

Table 4.1 Action steps to creating a welcoming environment *(continued)*

Action step	*Description*	*Example(s)*
3. Educate yourself regarding transgender-affirmative knowledge	• Be familiar with the history of the development of transgender and gender non-conforming identities. • Recognize the boundaries of your own competence. Seek ongoing educational opportunities. • Network with other knowledgeable community and national resources.	• *Read the recommended texts at the end of the chapters that are most relevant to your educational needs.* • *Consider your readiness to provide treatment in the context of your profession's ethical competence guidelines.* • *Seek out information from the Human Rights Campaign, Center of Excellence for Transgender Health, Transgender Europe (TGEU), The Transgender Project (Canada).*
4. Recognize Biases	• Examine your biases and beliefs regarding transgender individuals. • If you are committed to competence in terms of knowledge and self-awareness, and have experience in helping transgender clients in therapy, consider advertising your services.	• *Reflect on your history of working with transgender clients and re-read past clinical notes and documentation, if possible.* a. *Research implicit biases; some websites such as https://implicit.harvard.edu/implicit/ are available for this.* • *Research LGBT-friendly publications and websites that are specific to your area. Visit your practice website or profiles and look for signs that you present as an affirmative provider.*
5. Make appropriate modifications to your work	• Screen for health disparities and issues that might affect transgender clients without over pathologizing. • Recognize that societal bias disproportionately affects transgender individuals' access to services.	• *Knowing that there are elevated rates of suicidal thoughts and behaviors, or substance use, among transgender individuals increases the importance of asking about these issues at intake.* a. *When assessments are normed on gender, recognize that the measure may not be appropriate when working with transgender individuals.* • *Employment and housing discrimination may affect transgender clients and be able to assist with resources addressing these concerns.*

Identifying and Mitigating Bias in Health Care Service Provision

Many transgender individuals report instances of mistreatment and stigma in health care settings that are likely due to providers' lack of awareness of transgender issues. Due to understandable hesitations or fears, clients may possibly postpone or even forgo necessary care (Hughto, Reisner, & Pachankis, 2015). Other pressures also impact treatment-seeking: If a transgender individual chooses to physically transition using medical interventions, in many instances they must first be diagnosed with Gender Dysphoria and/or assessed for mental health conditions. Therefore, providers are often placed in the position of "gatekeeper" with regard to their clients' transition process. It is essential that the provider recognizes the inherently unequal balance of power in this relationship. It is also wise for a provider to acknowledge the potential effect this type of power differential may have with regards to a transgender client seeking or continuing care. A 21-year-old transman-identified individual illustrated this concern by stating, "*In the first few sessions I lied about a lot of things concerning my transition because I was afraid of gatekeeping.*"

Clients may be concerned about being pathologized, about the historical ambivalence toward medically transitioning versus socially transitioning, about being denied letters for hormone treatment or gender affirming surgeries, about being outed to insurance carriers or others, and about not "fitting the narrative" of what individuals believe is the archetypal transgender individual, among many other scenarios. These concerns were echoed in part by a 46-year-old non-binary transfeminine person: "*People wanted to make me fit into a gender binary. I have even been asked why I don't just commit to being '100% female' instead of staying in the middle. The therapist that said that was a cis[gender] lesbian. Goes to show that not all LGB people get it.*" We suggest having an up-front discussion on the effect gatekeeping may have on the relationship between the client and therapist to address any concerns a client may have and to diminish the power imbalance. In addition, there is value in respecting the client's identity, even when it does not fit with the mental health provider's anticipated identity goal.

It is paramount for mental health providers to be aware of the power they hold as professionals, and they need to be familiar with the effect anti-transgender prejudice (or transphobia) has on the lives of transgender individuals. Results from the 2015 U.S. Transgender Survey indicated that 23% of transgender individuals experienced some form of housing discrimination in the past year as a result of their transgender status, and over half of transgender individuals have been verbally harassed in a public place because of their transgender identity (James et al., 2016). Furthermore, a striking 55% of transgender individuals were denied medical coverage for transition-related necessities (Austin & Craig, 2015; James et al., 2016; for more detail see Chapter 2). An experience recounted by a 24-year-old, non-binary, transmasculine individual sheds light on the reality of these statistics: "*I was held in a mental health hospital involuntarily during my transition because of a suicide attempt related to dysphoria and was misgendered and referred to by my birth name frequently. I was also kept in a single room because they couldn't figure out what gender roommate to give me.*" Very recently, a 14-year-old transgender male committed suicide shortly after being treated at a Gender Management Clinic in San Diego, CA for anxiety and depression related to his gender identity. His family asserts that being consistently misgendered while in the hospital increased his dysphoria and may have led to his suicide (Bever, 2016).

Addressing Gaps in Your Knowledge Regarding Transgender Individuals' Experiences

One of the most commonly cited barriers to adequate mental health care is providers' lack of knowledge about transgender issues, ranging from ignorance about basic vocabulary to uncertainty about what transition might entail (Bauer et al., 2009; Dispenza & O'Hara, 2016; Goldberg, 2006; Johnson, Shipherd & Walton, 2015; Lucksted, 2004; Pitts, Couch, Mulcare, Croy, & Mitchell, 2009; Rutherford, McIntyre, Daley, & Ross, 2012). As a result, transgender clients often find themselves in the position of educating their providers about transgender experiences and their health care needs (Benson, 2013; Kidd, Veltman, Gately, Chan, & Cohen, 2011). Consequently, transgender clients often face an uphill battle when finding competent mental health and general health care providers who are not only sufficiently trained in transgender issues but also willing to do all that they can to facilitate a healthy transition in light of the geographic, financial, and interpersonal barriers to transition services (Benson, 2013). Transgender individuals often describe having to "doctor shop" in order to find a competent, passionate, and welcoming provider. A 48-year-old transguy describes his strategy for seeking specialized services: "*[I'm] currently seeing a great clinical psychologist who is knowledgeable and totally cool with gender and sexually diverse people. I deliberately sought out a place that specialized in minority groups.*" For those with a less productive search for a provider, though, this process can be frustrating and can discourage transgender individuals from seeking help altogether.

Providers should systematically assess their own competence regarding transgender issues regularly, as it is not always possible to know that gender identity issues will arise prior to taking on a client (Boroughs, Bedoya, O'Cleirigh, & Safren, 2015; Cochran & Robohm, 2015; Matza, Sloan, & Kauth, 2015). This is clearly not a one-time self-assessment for several reasons: The literature regarding transgender individuals is continually evolving, one's understanding of transgender issues increases substantially with experience, and biases may re-emerge at any time. As identified in the American Psychological Association's ethical standard 2.01 *Boundaries of Competence*, American psychologists must either "have or obtain the training, experience, consultation or supervision necessary to ensure the competence of their services" (American Psychological Association, 2010, p. 4). Likewise, the European Federation of Psychologists' Association's Meta-Code of Ethics standard 2.2 *Competence* states that European psychologists, "recognise the boundaries of their particular competencies and the limitations of their expertise. They provide only those services and use only those techniques for which they are qualified by education, training, or experience" (European Federation of Psychologists' Associations, 2005). Self-reflection regarding these standards will help mental health professionals to determine whether they are culturally competent and if they have the knowledge, awareness, and skills (Sue, Arredondo, & McDavis, 1992) to work with transgender clients. Referral may at times be the best decision for the client for various reasons and being able to provide an excellent referral is an important service. As one 30-year-old male indicated in our survey, "*I had to do some very deep research to make sure I was going to be going to a place that had professionals in this field.*" Of course, these clinical and cultural competence skills are always in development, especially with novice mental health professionals; but the best practice is to do the necessary homework to be "up-to-speed" with current standards, social climates, and the needs of the client.

As mentioned, transgender individuals who are seeking mental health services will be coming in for an array of reasons. It is important to know that many transgender individuals choose to socially transition (e.g., name change, pronoun change), while others may choose to physically transition (e.g., hormone treatment, gender affirming surgery); some may choose neither (Hughto, Reisner, & Pachankis, 2015). Each client should be treated as an individual, and providers must respect the client's decision regarding the degree to which they desire to transition. Some transgender individuals embrace certain terms in accordance with their gender identity or expression, such as *transgender woman*, *transgender man*, *genderqueer*, and *gender variant*, among many others (it is useful to note that "transgender*ed*" is a problematic term for various reasons; Benjamin, 1966; Hughto, Reisner, & Pachankis, 2015; King, Winter, & Webster, 2009; Tebbe, Moradi, & Ege, 2014). With knowledge of these nuances, it is critical to reflect on the language used by the provider, by other personnel (e.g., front office, billing staff), and in paperwork. Often, pronouns—in particular, being referred to by an undesired pronoun—are a major source of dysphoria or discomfort for many transgender individuals. Many of the respondents to our survey emphasized that they felt respected and affirmed when providers used their stated pronouns, and invalidated when they did not. A 21-year-old transmasculine individual responded, "*Always ask and use proper pronouns and names. Never assume the chart is right, always ask the person.*"

Many providers may be wary to ask about gender identity and expression at intake for fear of outing transgender individuals or making cisgender individuals feel awkward or confused. We recommend asking all clients these questions during intake and have responses ready for potentially awkward reactions. Being prepared for reactions will increase providers' comfort with routinely asking about gender identity. For example, a client might say, "*Why are you asking about that? Don't I look like a man?*" You might have a prepared response such as, "*Because not all aspects of someone's identity are visible, I ask all clients about their gender identity.*"

It is necessary to be respectful to clients while also following legal guidelines for billing and record keeping. For example, you have a client named Jackson who identifies as male, but you notice that his insurance card states that he is a "female" with the name "Tamara". Instances like this might require creativity in establishing a system in which you can maintain records based on Jackson's legal gender and name for billing purposes, while also noting his authentic name and gender identity so that agency staff do not misgender or incorrectly address him. However, make sure to communicate unique chart notation throughout the clinic to avoid outing and embarrassing the client and to also maintain consistency, privacy, and respect for the client's wishes. For example, a preferred name field and a gender identity field located near the top of the electronic record or physical chart offers an easy way to find this information. It is important for a provider to anticipate obstacles in billing, electronic patient records, and other structural systems before they occur. Do not wait for a client to discover these obstacles; do a preliminary check of your billing policies, insurance claims filing, and other systems for a mock client who identifies as transgender; and consider non-binary identifications in particular when examining record systems. Working with administrative staff on these issues to ensure that they can file appropriate claims while respecting clients' gender identity and expression will demonstrate a safe and understanding environment. Going through this exercise will help to routinize the experience for future clients and demonstrate your sensitivity as you inform them of how billing will be addressed.

It is also important to recognize that transgender individuals may not only seek services prior to their transition but also throughout or even years after. A 35-year-old transman brought up this concern in response to a question about negative experiences in the mental health field.

> *The barrier I'm up against is finding providers with experience in counseling clients who have already transitioned. I've tried people who flat out have no experience with trans individuals, although that may be more disappointing than negative. I had a therapist once who wanted me to blame my mother for all kinds of stuff, including not teaching me to be a 'proper girl.'*

In creating a welcoming environment, providers should, of course, be accepting of individuals at all stages of their transition. Therapists should also be aware that certain theoretical perspectives may automatically pathologize transgender individuals or their families; as illustrated in the quote above, some theoretical orientations may presuppose, for example, that transgender identities are rooted in family-of-origin conflicts, but there are no data to support such a position.

Overall, it is the duty of the clinic to create a space for a client to be who they are without any fear or reservations. Obtaining transgender affirmative knowledge will surely be noticed by your clients, however obvious or subtle you presume it to be. A 22-year-old, non-binary, trans individual picked up on their providers' knowledge and acceptance,

> *She referred me to a doctor to prescribe me hormones after just one meeting, after we discussed my transition-related needs and my readiness to start [hormones]. This stands out to me especially since many health care professionals do not consider non-binary people to be "as trans" as binary trans people, or consider non-binary folks' access to transition-related care to be as imperative.*

Furthermore, a 24-year-old woman also celebrated her providers' awareness: "*Absolutely. My therapist had plenty of experience working with the trans community and had plenty of connections, such as endocrinologists, laser [hair] removal, speech therapy, etc.*"

A Welcoming Clinic Environment Is Both Free of Bias and Overtly Affirming

Common biases that lay people and professionals might hold about transgender individuals include, but are not limited to, assuming that people only transition within the binary (e.g., only transition female-to-male or male-to-female) or that transgender individuals are less socially and mentally fit than cisgender individuals (Reed, Franks, & Scherr, 2015). Others may assume that the gender identity development process and coming out process are equivalent to that of sexual minorities or that transgender individuals are dangerous or threats to society (Feldman & Crandall, 2007). Examining one's own biases is crucial in establishing a welcoming environment.

Beyond being aware of blatant anti-transgender prejudices and recognizing the history of transgender people, mental health care providers should consider things that might stand out to a transgender client: How did they find out about your services (e.g., standard listing, transgender-friendly outlets, word-of-mouth)? What do your intake forms look like (e.g., binary options for gender or open-ended)? How are clients greeted by staff (e.g., friendly smiles versus confused looks or whispers about what their gender is)? What bathroom options are available (e.g., gender neutral or gendered stalls)? What in the physical environment signals that transgender people are expected and welcome here? Where are your services advertised (e.g., LGBT friendly outlets)? Through this exercise, it becomes apparent that there are several steps that can be taken to present a welcome and safe space for a transgender client. Several small changes may help to indicate inclusivity without disrupting the overall space. Suggestions include posting a Pride flag (note: There is a specific transgender Pride flag in addition to the ubiquitous LGBT Pride rainbow flag) or other signs and symbols that indicate allies' support (e.g., safe zone stickers). Also, making available magazines that represent gender identities outside of the cisgender binary (e.g., FTM magazine), business cards of community providers who are LGBT friendly, and pamphlets of resources for other safe spaces (e.g., Trevor Project, Human Rights Campaign) sends a positive message. Although these changes are small, they represent symbols of support, respect, and recognition of the transgender community. However, it is vital that these symbols of a safe environment are also supported by a therapeutic alliance that is genuinely affirming and free of bias or judgment.

Digging Deeper: Addressing Subtle and Implicit Biases

As it has become less socially appropriate to express overtly negative attitudes towards transgender individuals, it is important to consider the ways in which subtle or overt biases may still linger in mental health care settings. Transphobia and its effect on mental health care delivery can be understood on two levels—explicitly (when the bias is readily identifiable, as we have described) as well as implicitly. Implicit attitudes can be thought of as relatively automatic and ingrained; they occur even without our awareness and can escape our attention (Spruyt & Moors, 2009). For example, although a provider may not feel negatively towards transgender individuals, they may be quick to label transgender clients as depressed because of assumptions about their clients' experiences, or they may assume that transgender clients' distress is always rooted in a diagnosis of Gender Dysphoria. This concern is echoed by a 21-year-old transman-identified individual in our survey: "*They [providers] need to realize that dysphoria is not required to be transgender nor are they [transgender individuals] making it up.*" These relatively automatic judgments have the potential to significantly affect treatment decisions. Research suggests that health care providers do, in fact, have implicit biases against racial (Green et al., 2007; Sabin, Rivara, & Greenwald, 2008) and sexual (Burke et al., 2015; Cochran, Peavy, & Cauce, 2008) minorities. These implicit biases have been shown to have real-life treatment implications that can negatively affect the services a client receives. In one study of medical providers, Green and colleagues (2007) demonstrated that doctors were more likely to prescribe medication to a White patient, rather than to a Black patient who was presenting with the same symptoms. Even after explicit biases were controlled for, implicit biases alone were correlated with treatment differences. In other words, even in the absence of explicit biases, implicit attitudes can affect the course of treatment and may be outside of the provider's awareness. Thus, working in a system that includes the opportunity for professional consultation is important for checking one's implicit biases.

Analogous research has not been conducted with the consideration of transgender clients. While explicit transphobia is easier to spot and address, implicit biases have proven to be subtle and enduring (Devine, Forscher, Austin, & Cox, 2012). Thus, it is mental health providers' responsibility to understand the way implicit biases function and how they may be affecting their work with transgender individuals.

In addition to the implicit biases mentioned above, consider what other assumptions you may have about transgender clients. Do you assume that family or partners will be less (or more) supportive of transitioning than they might actually be? Is it possible that you might inadvertently treat a transgender client as more fragile than others, knowing that the person likely has experienced discrimination? Are you adjusting your expectations regarding a client's capabilities or mental health status on the person being transgender? Are you comparing your own journey of identity development to theirs? This process of self-analysis may reveal important information as you strive to create a welcoming clinical environment for transgender clients.

Be Mindful of the Experiences of Specific Groups of Transgender Individuals

It is important for mental health care professionals to recognize that not all clients who are transgender share the same experiences. While the current Gender Dysphoria diagnosis was an attempt to encompass individual differences in the experience of dysphoria, there is not an adequate distinction between social dysphoria (or discomfort regarding the ways that others read one's gender in a social context) and physical dysphoria (or discomfort regarding the ways that one experiences their gender in a bodily sense). Likewise, researchers generally lump transgender individuals together and do not publish on the experiences of specific gender identities. This has the potential to "blur the lines" between the experiences of diverse gender identities encompassed within the transgender umbrella, which may in turn create generalized expectations of what it means to be transgender. In addition, transgender men and women and non-binary individuals may have unique gendered experiences regarding transition, identity disclosure, and interpersonal trauma. For example, transition procedures, costs, and availability vary for transgender men and transgender women, and many transgender individuals may not desire or be able to afford such procedures.

While the majority of research on transgender-related issues focuses on gender binary identities, only a fraction of LGBT research and practice guidelines address the particular issues and experiences of non-binary individuals. Given the lack of transgender-related knowledge that providers endorse, the dearth of educational resources for mental health providers on individuals with non-binary gender identities offers a dim outlook for the field's working competencies for this population (Boroughs et al, 2015; Cochran & Robohm, 2015; Matza, Sloan, & Kauth, 2015). By avoiding gender binary assumptions in written and verbal language, mental health settings allow more space for clients to express their authentic selves and lived experiences.

Elderly transgender individuals may face specific challenges that are important to consider in providing care. Depending on the age at which the individual transitioned (if applicable), family members affected by the process may include multiple generations, with often complicated relationships with the client. Being out may be similarly more complicated, as older people are likely to have met friends, acquaintances, and coworkers at various stages of life. Planning for long-term care becomes more complex, as few long-term care facilities provide transgender-friendly environments. Later-life issues such as reappraisal of life's meaning and consideration of regrets may include additional layers, such as not transitioning earlier in life and not having been able to live authentically.

Importantly, intersecting identities such as class, race, sexual orientation, and disability status influence transgender individuals' likelihood of seeking treatment as well as their experiences once they access mental health services. Fears and lived experiences regarding the ways in which certain identities—particularly ethnicity—might jointly increase the odds for discrimination can discourage multiply-marginalized transgender individuals from seeking health care services. Barriers to care for transgender individuals with additional minority identities can vary depending on mounting stigmas, financial resources, and community values (Nemoto, Operario, & Keatley, 2008). For more on intersectionality of identities, see Chapter 3.

Beyond identities such as race, disability status, and age, providers and staff should also examine their biases about stigmatized experiences such as substance use disorders, sex work history, and HIV-positive status. The likelihood of these experiences is increased by the health disparities discussed in Chapter 3, and mitigating biases against these experiences is important to enacting a welcoming clinic environment.

Adapt These Suggestions to Your Specific Setting

Understanding the experience of transgender clients includes recognizing the broader sociopolitical context in which you live. Policies and practices at the level of your country, region, city or town, and neighborhood all affect transgender individuals' sense of belongingness (or lack thereof). Individuals who are transgender might be dissuaded from seeking care or disclosing their gender identity based on both present and historical factors unique to certain care settings. Providers should be aware of their agencies' specific resources, bathroom accessibility, room accommodations (if applicable), and non-discrimination policies that might apply to transgender clients.

Certain settings, more than others, may be perceived as less affirming for individuals who are transgender. While agencies should be proactive in advertising their acceptance and celebration of gender diversity, mental health care settings with more obvious histories or perceptions of stigmatization should make these messages particularly visible. For example, the U.S. military's history of discharging, denying benefits to, and silencing the identities of transgender service members could engender the perception that Veteran Health Administration (VHA) facilities today are not welcoming places for gender minority veterans. Indeed, this history is likely evident in recent research in which only around one-third of VHA providers and clients rated the VHA setting as being *somewhat* or *very welcoming* to veterans who are transgender (Sherman et al., 2014). On the other hand, as Kauth and Shipherd (2016) indicate, many VHA facilities have recently been recognized for their LGBT inclusivity. Still, negative perceptions may be resistant to change, even if improvements in training and acceptance have been made at that health care setting (for more detail see Chapter 2).

In both integrated and co-located health care settings such as national/federal or state health care facilities, medical centers, and academic health centers, shared health records warrant explicit communication about how gender identity information is documented and shared. To respect clients' wishes about their degree of identity disclosure, providers should inform their clients about who has access to their gender identity information, how this information is used, as well as the clients' rights in terms of confidentiality. The client should also feel safe in knowing that everyone with access to the shared health record has an acceptable amount of competency for working with transgender clients; thus, training should be made accessible for everyone who will have access to clients' gender identity information (Callahan et al., 2014). The issues presented by a shared record warrant a conversation about confidentiality and best care practices that are facilitated by having gender identity information open to all practitioners.

Finally, in settings where mental health care is delivered in part or completely in group format, such as some inpatient settings or substance use agencies, the provider only has limited control over the environment, as other clients' attitudes toward transgender individuals are frequently unknown. Other clients may have a negative reaction to a transgender client's identity or may make explicitly transphobic comments in session. Providers should work to minimize negative experiences that may happen in group work by establishing a commitment to inclusivity that includes gender identity and expression at the start of all groups, by serving as advocates for the rights of transgender people, and by addressing instances of bias or discrimination directly.

In sum, providing a welcoming clinic environment for transgender clients is not just commensurate with the WPATH *Standards of Care*, it is in keeping with the principles and values of all mental health professions. We feel it is fitting to end with the words of a 25-year-old man who participated in our survey: "*Being treated equally makes you feel like a normal person and not an outsider.*"

Take Home Points:

- Providers must recognize the historical legacy of mental health systems regarding transgender individuals.
- A welcoming environment cannot be achieved unless providers and staff take the perspective of a transgender individual seeking treatment at their agency or facility.
- Considering one's ability to provide a welcoming environment requires an appraisal of one's competence, including relevant knowledge and an ongoing examination of explicit and implicit biases.

Recommended Readings

American Psychological Association (2015). Guidelines for psychological practice with transgender and gender non-conforming people. *American Psychologist*,

70(9), 832–864. Retrieved from https://www.apa.org/practice/guidelines/transgender.pdf

Deustch, M. B. (Ed.). (2016). *Guidelines for the primary and gender-affirming care of transgender and gender nonbinary people.* Center of Excellence for Transgender Health. Retrieved from http://transhealth.ucsf.edu/pdf/Transgender-PGACG-6-17-16.pdf

Lev, A. I. (2004). *Transgender emergence: Therapeutic guidelines for working with gender-variant people and their relatives.* Binghamton, NY: Haworth Press.

Sallans, R. (2012). *Second son: Transitioning toward my destiny, love, and life.* Green Bay, WI: Title Town Publishing.

References

American Psychological Association. (2010). Ethical principles of psychologists and code of conduct. Washington, DC: Author. Retrieved from www.apa.org/ethics/code/index.aspx

Austin, A., & Craig, S. L. (2015). Transgender affirmative cognitive behavioral therapy: Clinical considerations and applications. *Professional Psychology: Research and Practice, 46*(1), 21–29.

Bauer, G. R., Hammond, R., Travers, R., Kaay, M., Hohenadel, K. M., & Boyce, M. (2009). "I don't think this is theoretical; this is our lives": How erasure impacts health care for transgender people. *Journal of the Association of Nurses in AIDS Care, 20*(5), 348–361.

Benjamin, H. (1966). *The transsexual phenomenon.* New York, NY: The Julian Press. Retrieved from www.mut23.de/texte/Harry%20Benjamin%20-%20The%20Transsexual%20Phenomenon.pdf

Benson, K. E. (2013). Seeking support: Transgender client experiences with mental health services. *Journal of Feminist Family Therapy, 25*(1), 17–40.

Bever, L. (2016). Transgender boy's mom sues hospital, saying he 'went into spiral' after staff called him a girl. *The Washington Post.* Retrieved from https://www.washingtonpost.com/news/to-your-health/wp/2016/10/03/mother-sues-hospital-for-discrimination-after-staff-kept-calling-her-transgender-son-a-girl/

Boroughs, M. S., Bedoya, C. A., O'Cleirigh, C., & Safren, S. A. (2015). Toward defining, measuring, and evaluating LGBT cultural competence for psychologists. *Clinical Psychology: Science and Practice, 22,* 151–171.

Burke, S. E., Dovidio, J. F., Przedworski, J. M., Hardeman, R. R., Perry, S. P., . . . & van Ryn, M. (2015). Do contact and empathy mitigate bias against gay and lesbian people among first-year medical students? A report from the medical student CHANGE study. *Academic Medicine, 90*(5), 645–651.

Callahan, E. J., Sitkin, N., Ton, H., Eidson-Ton, S., Weckstein, J., & Latimore, D. (2014). Introducing sexual orientation and gender identity into the electronic health record: One academic health center's experience. *Academic Medicine, 90*(2), 154–160.

Cochran, B. N., Peavy, K. M., & Cauce, A. M. (2008). Substance abuse treatment providers' explicit and implicit attitudes regarding sexual minorities. *Journal of Homosexuality, 53*(3), 181–207.

Cochran, B. N., & Robohm, J. S. (2015). Integrating LGBT competencies into the multicultural curriculum of graduate psychology training programs: Expounding and expanding upon Hope and Chappell's choice points: Commentary on "Extending training in multicultural competencies to include individuals identifying as lesbian, gay, and bisexual: Key choice points for clinical psychology training programs." *Clinical Psychology Science and Practice, 22,* 119–126.

Devine, P. G., Forscher, P. S., Austin, A. J., & Cox, W. T. L. (2012). Long-term reduction in implicit race bias: A prejudice habit-breaking intervention. *Journal of Experimental Social Psychology, 48,* 1267–1278.

Dispenza, F., & O'Hara, C. (2016). Correlates of transgender and gender non-conforming counseling competencies among psychologists and mental health practitioners. *Psychology of Sexual Orientation and Gender Diversity, 3*(2), 156–164.

European Federation of Psychologists' Associations. (2005). Meta-code of ethics. Retrieved from www.bdp-verband.org/bdp/verband/clips/efpa_metacode_en.pdf

Feldman, D. B., & Crandall, C. S. (2007). Dimensions of mental illness stigma: What about mental illness causes social rejection? *Journal of Social and Clinical Psychology, 26,* 137–154.

Goldberg, J. M. (2006). Training community-based clinicians in transgender care. *International Journal of Transgenderism, 9*(3–4), 219–231.

Green, A. R., Carney, D. R., Pallin, D. J., Ngo, L. H., Raymond, K. L., . . . & Banaji, M. R. (2007). Implicit bias among physicians and its prediction of thrombolysis decisions for black and white patients. *Journal of General Internal Medicine, 22*(9), 1231–1238.

Hirschfeld, M., & Schmidt, W. J. (1923/1984). Die intersexuelle konstitution. *Jahrbuch fur Sexuelle Zwischenstufen.* Frankfurt am Main: Qumran.

Hughto, J. M. W., Reisner, S. L., & Pachankis, J. E. (2015). Transgender stigma and health: A critical review of stigma determinants, mechanisms, and interventions. *Social Science & Medicine, 147,* 222–231.

James, S. E., Herman, J. L., Rankin, S., Keisling, M., Mottet, L., & Anafi, M. (2016). *The Report of the 2015 U.S. Transgender Survey.* Washington, DC: National Center for Transgender Equality. Retrieved from www.transequality.org/sites/default/files/docs/USTS-Full-Report-FINAL.PDF

Johnson, L., Shipherd, J. C. & Walton, H. (2016). The psychologist's role in transgender-specific care with U.S. veterans. *Psychological Services, 13*(1), 69–76.

Kauth, M. R., & Shipherd, J. C. (2016). Transforming a system: Improving patient-centered care for sexual and gender minority veterans. *LGBT Health, 3,* 177–179.

Kidd, S. A., Veltman, A., Gately, C., Chan, K. J., & Cohen, J. N. (2011). Lesbian, gay, and transgender persons with severe mental illness: Negotiating wellness in the context of multiple sources of stigma. *American Journal of Psychiatric Rehabilitation, 14*(1), 13–39.

King, M. E., Winter, S., & Webster, B. (2009). Contact reduces transprejudice: A study on attitudes towards transgenderism and transgender civil rights in Hong Kong. *International Journal of Sexual Health, 21*(1), 17–34.

Lucksted, A. (2004). Lesbian, gay, bisexual, and transgender people receiving services in the public mental health system: Raising issues. *Journal of Gay & Lesbian Psychotherapy, 8*(3–4), 25–42.

Matza, A. R., Sloan, C. A., & Kauth, M. R. (2015). Quality LGBT health education: A review of core reports and webinars. *Clinical Psychology: Science and Practice, 22,* 127–144.

Nemoto, T., Operario, D., & Keatley, J. (2008). Health and social services for male-to-female transgender persons of color in San Francisco. *International Journal of Transgenderism, 8*(2–3), 5–19.

Pitts, M. K., Couch, M., Mulcare, H., Croy, S., & Mitchell, A. (2009). Transgender people in Australia and New Zealand: Health, well-being, and access to health services. *Feminism & Psychology, 19*(4), 475–495.

Reed, O. M., Franks, A. S., & Scherr, K. C. (2015). Are perceptions of transgender individuals affected by mental illness stigma? A moderated mediation analysis of anti-transgender prejudice in hiring recommendations. *Psychology of Sexual Orientation and Gender Diversity, 2*(4), 463–469.

Rutherford, K., McIntyre, J., Daley, A., & Ross, L. E. (2012). Development of expertise in mental health service provision for lesbian, gay, bisexual, and transgender communities. *Medical Education, 46*(9), 903–913.

Sabin, J. A., Rivara, F. P., & Greenwald, A. G. (2008). Physician implicit attitudes and stereotypes about race and quality of medical care. Medical Care, *46*(7), 678–685.

Santayana, G. (1905). *The life of reason or the phases of human progress (One-volume edition).* New York, NY: Charles Scribner's Sons.

Sherman, M. D., Kauth, M. R., Ridener, L., Shipherd, J. C., Bratkovich, K., & Beaulieu, G. (2014). An empirical investigation of challenges and recommendations for welcoming sexual and gender minority veterans into VA care. *Professional Psychology: Research and Practice, 45*(6), 433–442.

Spruyt, A., & Moors, A. (2009). Implicit measures: A normative analysis and review. *Psychological Bulletin, 135*(3), 347–368.

Sue, D.W., Arredondo, P., McDavis, R. (1992). Multicultural counseling competencies and standards: a call to the profession. *Journal of Counseling & Development, 70*, 477–486.

Tebbe, E. A., Moradi, B., & Ege, E. (2014). Revised and abbreviated forms of the genderism and transphobia scale: Tools for assessing anti-transgender prejudice. *Journal of Counseling Psychology, 61*(4), 581–592.

5 Supporting the Transgender Individual in Deciding Their Pathway

Ruben A. Hopwood, MDiv, PhD

Gender identity is not static or fixed and has fluidity across the lifespan. Gender identities may not align fully or comfortably with a person's sex as assigned at birth. Though a binary system remains the dominant narrative and expectation amongst most cultures (Chang, Singh, & Rossman, 2017; Enke, 2016), gender identity may be more clearly understood as a type of continuum, spectrum, or constellation comprised of many overlapping personality traits and aptitudes, each of which may be categorized as more or less masculine or feminine, according to particular cultures and customs.

The common assumption and expectation since at least the 1930s (Meyerowitz, 2002) has been that persons for whom their sex assigned at birth does not align with their experienced and espoused gender should move along a linear and binary pathway to total hormonal and surgical reassignment to the opposite end of a male–female binary existence (Beek, Kreukels, Cohen-Kettenis, & Steensma, 2015). Discrimination against gender diverse people combined with a forced conformity of cultural conceptual frameworks of only binary gender options has historically caused many transgender individuals significant life challenges and psychological distress (James et al., 2016; Iantaffi & Bockting, 2011; Mizock & Fleming, 2011; Mizock & Mueser, 2014). It is the job of mental health professionals to help transgender individuals alleviate this distress and support exploration and working out of life challenges.

Historically, mental health professionals have played a central role in the process of transgender people who sought gender affirming treatments (Bockting, Knudson, & Goldberg, 2007). That role has often felt unsupportive and uninformed and experienced as "gatekeeping"; imposing decisions as to who was appropriate or "ready" for medical treatment (McLemore, 2015; Singh & Burnes, 2010; Siverskog, 2014). This gatekeeping function has often served to enforce gender binaries and encourage transition pathways that fit medical models of traditional (i.e., gender binary) transgender care, even when this was not the goal of the individual (Chang et al., 2017). To move away from gatekeeping, the provider should work to suspend assumptions as they listen, explore, and guide transgender clients regarding possibilities, risks, and potential outcomes along their pathways to integration of an internal and external sense of self (American Psychological Association, 2015; Bockting et al., 2007; Burnes et al., 2010; Wylie et al., 2014).

The mental health professional's role in gender affirmation is increasingly interdisciplinary and consultative with medical professionals who prescribe hormone treatments, or who perform gender affirming surgical procedures. The overall work of the mental health provider in treating transgender clients involves facilitating the client's exploration and integration of their gender (for additional detail on one approach to this work, readers are referred to Chapter 8). This role is accomplished through the ability to discover and explore the specific details, needs, and desires of the person seeking treatment in order to offer appropriate, relevant, and non-discriminatory options, interventions, referrals, and supports (American Psychological Association, 2015; World Professional Association for Transgender Health, 2011). Mental health professionals may be called upon to offer counseling that explores gender or other concurrent life issues to assist the client in determining goals and optimal pathways for gender affirmation or expression, and to assess and provide professional comments on readiness and eligibility for specific treatments. To perform these functions, mental health professionals need to be aware of several issues that may affect gender identity and presentation, influence treatment options, and shape probable outcomes in choosing and pursuing a particular pathway toward gender affirmation or clarification.

This chapter addresses the primary question of how to support and enable transgender clients to determine their own best pathway toward gender affirmation and expression. The chapter elucidates common transition-related psychological, social, and cultural concerns of transgender people and provides a basic outline for assessing gender dysphoria along with readiness and eligibility for gender affirming medical treatments, with the aim of supporting the client in fully internalizing and integrating their gender identity into their life. What this chapter does not offer is a simple, singular, or "right" way to approach supporting gender diverse people.

Support of Gender Affirmation Goals

Clinical support of transgender people is inherently interdisciplinary. Supports need to be client-centered, taking into consideration as primary factors the client's individual desires, needs, and situation. Knowledge of non-binary as well as binary gender affirmation pathways will help providers reduce their assumptions of what a gender affirmation pathway "should" look like and will leave room for considering multiple options for affirmation that fit each individual more accurately. This broad and open approach avoids the pitfall of directing people into unwanted binary trajectories (Wylie et al., 2014).

In order to access needed supports and services, a transgender person may need a diagnosis of Gender Dysphoria on which to base some if not all the treatments sought. However, the diagnosis itself may be seen by transgender clients as part of the pathologizing cultural environment that produces distress. The issue of making Gender Dysphoria a diagnosis remains a heated topic without a simple or unified answer at this point in time (Drescher, 2014; Rettew, 2012).

While acknowledging the complicated relationship and historical context mental health professionals and transgender people have with the diagnosis of Gender Dysphoria in the DSM-5 and Gender Identity Disorder in the ICD-10-CM, the purpose of this chapter is not to debate these controversies. This chapter discusses Gender Dysphoria broadly and when the diagnosis may be appropriate as well as beneficial in providing documentation for medically necessary treatment.

Any treatment needs to be informed by current guidelines and recommendations for care of the population (American Psychological Association, 2015; Bhasin, Safer, & Tangpricha, 2009; Burnes et al., 2010; World Professional Association for Transgender Health, 2011) as well as employing the necessary supervision for monitoring and identifying the provider's biases and assumptions in the care provided or recommended (Boroughs, Bedoya, O'Cleirigh, & Safren, 2015; Burnes et al., 2010). Treatment should aim to neither impede nor encourage any specific outcome, but support the client in making their own best choices using the best information available at the time.

In clinical work, the provider needs to do the following:

- Suspend any assumptions of the client's desired goals and outcomes. Resist the assumption that a more socially normative gender identity or expression is equivalent to better mental health and well-being. Consult the client first about goals and identity and include the client in any treatment planning and recommendations. Support the client in articulating and defining their gender experience and how best to express it and move toward integration and comfort with their gender as it is. This includes acting on the premise that individuals have the capacity to consent to treatment and life choices unless there is a concern about capacity to make medical decisions (e.g., in the case of advanced Alzheimer's disease or other cognitive limitations).
- Determine the client's focus for treatment at the initial encounter and assess all life areas (e.g., work, family, social, etc.), not just gender identity. Avoid proscriptive treatment approaches, and use the client's priorities and situation to inform the structure or trajectory and timing of treatment. Start treatment and supports based on the client's priorities, neither asking the client to go back to previous stages of development to "prove" themselves or catch the provider up to them, nor rushing the client forward to another developmental stage before they are emotionally and systemically able to manage the changes in their lives. Remain flexible and support the client as they progress, even if they pause or change direction in their goals. Transition goals and pathways are not always linear, and there is no reason to insist that the client move in one direction or continue down one pathway to some preconceived end once started.

- Present well-informed information and guidance about gender affirmation options, both medical and non-medical, at the level needed for the client to comprehend the information. Options should include gender confirming as well as gender nullification treatments (i.e., removing all externally visible genitals so the body is literally "neutral" in appearance). Discuss risks and effects of all options being considered in an unbiased manner without unduly influencing the choices the client makes. Introduce gender-appropriate affirmation and protective options that the client may be unaware of, such as body contouring prosthetics or devices, reproductive preservation options, vocal and behavioral coaching and grooming services (see Chapter 10 for additional information), and various surgical (Chapter 9) and hormonal treatments (Chapter 6). To do this effectively and competently, the provider must engage in continuing self-education in transgender treatment and gender affirmation options through consultation, courses, conferences, and reading current clinical literature in these topics.
- Assess your client's understanding of risks and benefits for the gender affirmation pathway chosen and explore possible social and physical effects and risks of those choices. Take special care to explore and facilitate provision of information and consultations with medical providers on medical or surgical body modification risks and effects when appropriate. (The reader is directed to further consult the chapters on hormone treatment [Chapter 6] and surgeries [Chapter 9] to assist with guidance on these areas of treatment.)
- Assess and facilitate non-clinical supports for transgender clients. There are various supports in addition to mental health professional supports that will enhance the outcomes and overall well-being of transgender persons. These supports include peer supports and mentoring, ability to contribute to one's community, family support and affirmation, community support in general, supportive work and housing environments, and participation in and belonging to religious and spiritual communities that are supportive of the individual.
- Establish and use a network of interdisciplinary providers and specialists to offer consultation, supervision, and expertise outside the provider's own scope or capacity in support of clients' goals. These specialists may include primary care providers, speech and language professionals, endocrinologists, surgeons, reproductive specialists, dermatology, substance treatment specialists, case management, voice coaches, electrologists, lawyers, domestic violence and homeless services, immigration, etc. Coordinate services as needed to support the client's attainment of goals for gender affirmation or collaborate with the professional who is coordinating services and support for the client.
- Assess for co-occurring mental health and medical issues and confer with other mental health and medical providers to understand any serious mental illness and/or medical issues the client may be managing (see also

Chapter 7). Explore how these issues may interact with or affect gender affirmation and expression for the individual, as well as identity formation and consolidation, and the ability to engage in self-care. For example, a mental health provider can assist in smoking cessation, weight loss or nutritional issues, medication adherence and other behavioral change goals that can reduce or eliminate barriers to gender affirming medical treatments. Co-occurring mental health conditions and responses to stress demonstrate the consistent course and prognosis as fitting the diagnosis regardless of gender identity. Some gender affirming treatments, however, may trigger a destabilization of symptoms, such as the depressive effects possible with estrogen treatments. These shifts in mental health should not be construed as an indication of gender affirming treatment being in error, or regret, and should not be used as a rationale for stopping gender affirming treatment without clear and compelling clinical cause. That said, additional supports and interventions may be indicated.

- Engage the client in self-examination and exploration of their definitions and expectations of gender (e.g., what it means to be a man; a woman) as it impacts their own lives and trajectories. Include examination and assessment of body discomfort and body dysmorphic concerns and expectations, particularly for those seeking medical interventions. For example, does the client hold unrealistic ideals of what it means to be a man or a woman? Alternatively, is there a belief that transition will solve all struggles and conflicts or is there an appreciation that transitioning will include its own challenges?
- Assess experiences of and impact from discrimination, oppression, stigma, and trauma on the individual's experience and expression of their gender and their access to or barriers to care and treatment of any kind. For instance, in the United States (U.S.) transgender individuals experience three times higher rates of unemployment (15%; U.S. rate is 5%), increased workplace discrimination due to gender identity (30%), high lifetime rates of sexual assault (47% transgender; rates of rape for U.S. cisgender women are 18.3%; for U.S. cisgender men, 1.4%; rates of other sexual violence in the U.S. for cisgender women and men are 5.6% and 5.3%, respectively) (Centers for Disease Control, 2017). Rates worldwide for sexual violence against women range from 6.2% to 46.7% (World Health Organization, 2017). Rates of lifetime sexual assault for cisgender gay, bisexual, and lesbian adults in the U.S. range from 11.8% to 54.0% in men and 15.6% to 85.0% in women (Rothman, Exner, & Baughman, 2011), and very high rates of attempted suicide (40%; U.S. rate is 4.6%). (For further information on experiences of transgender people in the U.S., the reader is directed to James et al., 2016.) Many transgender individuals may experience posttraumatic stress as a result of severe discrimination and violence due to their gender. Reported rates of discrimination due to being perceived as transgender in the European Union are about 54% among transgender adults (European Union

Agency for Fundamental Rights, 2014); rates in the U.S. vary from 77% of transgender K–12 students reporting harassment and violence to 24% to 46% of transgender adults experiencing various types of harassment and violence (James et al., 2016). Given that a core feature of posttraumatic stress disorder (PTSD) is avoidance and hypervigilance to threat, it is important to recognize if the transition goals are primarily driven by a desire for reducing future risk of trauma. Treatment for PTSD and other sequelae of trauma and discrimination (e.g., anxiety, depression, substance abuse) might be necessary prior to fully understanding the transition goals without the potentially confounding effects of other symptoms. Advocate for clients as needed and appropriate. Assure that providers recommended as referrals are willing and competent to see transgender individuals or willing to receive education and guidance to increase their competence and their staff in service to these individuals.

- Prepare through education and supervision to perform assessments and provide referrals for medically necessary treatments when appropriate and desired. The following section will briefly address assessing readiness for medical gender affirmation treatments of hormones and surgeries.

Assessing Readiness for Medical Gender Treatments

Mental health providers are often called upon to provide professional opinions and referral letters for transgender people seeking medical interventions to modify their bodies for gender affirmation (Lev, 2009; World Professional Association for Transgender Health, 2011). In consideration of space constraints, this chapter will only broadly address the mental health provider's role in determining readiness for medically necessary treatments. The principles are similar for those who are seeking either gender affirming surgical procedures or hormone treatments, though hormone treatment is at least partially reversible, while surgical modification of the body is seen as having a permanent outcome. In all instances, whether medical or non-medical options are considered, the mental health professional may be called upon to assess whether the client broadly understands the repercussions of gender expression and/or affirmation choices they make given their unique circumstances. In order to assess the client's readiness, the provider must be adequately informed about medical interventions such as hormone treatments and surgical interventions to determine the client's level of realistic expectations and offer corrective information where needed. For an in-depth discussion of hormone treatments (Chapter 6) and surgical procedures (Chapter 9), the reader is directed to these respective chapters in this book.

Hormones

Hormonal treatments involve potential risks that must be discussed with any person seeking these treatments. Nearly 80% of transgender people in the

U.S. report that they desire hormone treatments, however, less than half (49%) report being able to access this treatment (James et al., 2016). In Europe, one report indicates that 39% of transgender people seek medical and psychological care and 18% go outside their country to access medical treatment (European Union Agency for Fundamental Rights, 2014). Transgender people who identify their gender identity more along a binary are more likely to desire hormone therapy (95%) compared to a smaller proportion of non-binary identified individuals (49%) (James et al., 2016). These distinctions play an important role in the mental health provider's assessment and ability to anticipate possible differences in the pathways that individual clients may want or need. Whenever possible, it is recommended that the mental health professional be in active communication with the prescribing provider during any assessment period and, ideally, during initial hormonal treatment as well. The following areas need to be assessed by the mental health provider prior to recommending hormone treatments:

- Clear indication of the medical necessity for the recommended feminizing/masculinizing treatment. The person meets criteria for Gender Dysphoria or is experiencing some type of clinical distress or functional impairments for which gender affirming hormonal treatment is indicated and likely to provide significant relief and/or improvement in functioning in everyday life.
- The individual has the capacity to understand the risks and effects of the treatment they seek and is legally able to give consent, or a guardian(s) can consent while the individual gives assent in the case of adults with cognitive or developmental delays.
- Co-occurring mental health and/or medical issues are reasonably well controlled and effects on these conditions from hormone treatments have been considered. Mental health issues by themselves rarely preclude hormone treatment. Mental health issues, such as depression, may improve after initiating some hormone treatments (Murad et al., 2010; White Hughto & Reisner, 2016). Co-occurring conditions that may be adversely affected by hormones during initiation of treatment (e.g., high blood pressure, cardiovascular disease, serious mental illness, psychosis, PTSD) should be adequately evaluated and determined to be stable for a reasonable amount of time prior to initiating hormone treatments. Some professionals recommend ongoing short-term supports from a mental health provider during hormone initiation in order to offer timely intervention should a mental health or medical condition become temporarily destabilized.
- Any substance use issues are reasonably well controlled. Substance use is prevalent within transgender populations and is often a symptom of ineffective coping that may respond positively to gender affirmation therapies (Sperber, Landers, & Lawrence, 2005). While safety and harm reduction approaches to substance and alcohol abuse may be necessary prior to hormonal or surgical treatments, expectations of total sobriety

may reflect a poor understanding of the stressors that the individual is managing and may exacerbate the person's distress. When substance abuse and addiction treatment is needed, it may also take extra work by the provider to locate transgender-competent substance treatment programs (Lombardi & van Servellen, 2000).

- Assess the individual's social supports and likelihood of following through with recommended treatments. Be cautious of biases and conceptualizations about what constitutes adequate supports. Some transgender people have meaningful online support systems while having only minimal in-person supports. Online support communities may allow people to express their gender identities in safe, empowering, and authentic ways in a manner not possible or even risky in person. Religious and spiritual communities may offer support, especially for older transgender populations (Porter, Ronneberg, & Witten, 2013). Supports may be quite different between communities based on gender identity and vary significantly between transgender men, transgender women, and non-binary individuals as well as between different races (Factor & Rothblum, 2008; James et al., 2016). Housing is part of assuring a safe environment for transition. Homelessness is not uncommon among transgender people and not a contraindication for starting hormones, although it can make compliance more complicated (Crossley, 2015; James et al., 2016). Facilitate connections to housing services and supports as needed, with the understanding that there are increased barriers to finding safe housing for transgender people (Reisner et al., 2014). Avoid delaying treatment to a person based solely on their housing status.

Surgeries

Surgery perhaps more so than hormones poses risks to the individual physically and psychologically and may offer significant benefits as well, depending on the individual's pathway to self-expression of gender. Surgical procedures to affirm, or confirm, a client's gender fall into two general categories—genital and non-genital. (There are myriad gender affirmation surgeries and the reader is referred to Chapter 9 and the larger literature for more in-depth descriptions and information on these various procedures.)

For the mental health professional, it is helpful to be familiar with common surgical procedures as well as postsurgical care plans and potential complications. A basic understanding is necessary to adequately evaluate realistic or distorted expectations a client may have about such interventions and help clients explore how the surgically altered aspects of their body will affect their social, psychological, spiritual or religious, and interpersonal lives. It is also necessary to have a basic understanding of the recovery and ongoing care needed for various surgical sites as the provider supports the client in making adequate preparations.

Not all transgender people want or have access (e.g., medical contraindications; absence of health insurance coverage; uncontrolled mental health issues, etc.) and financial ability to pursue surgeries. Desire or need for gender affirming surgeries differs across gender identities. Seeking gender affirming surgeries is also affected by life situations and external factors. It is important to recognize that not wanting surgical intervention does not equate to a lack of conviction about transition and is a valid choice. Transgender men are more likely to have gender affirmation surgeries (42%) than transgender women (28%) or non-binary individuals (9%) (James, et al., 2016). Complex medical comorbidities may also prevent clients from being able to access surgical interventions. Poverty can affect the pathway chosen by people and whether they can access costly procedures such as surgery (when they want it) and recover safely from the procedures afterwards. Economic as well as medical and mental health concerns need to be considered when assessing readiness for surgical procedures and self-care during and after these treatments.

Assessment for surgical readiness is very similar to the above hormone assessment, with some differences and additional exploration. As with hormones, individuals seeking surgeries need to have any co-occurring mental health and medical conditions well controlled and stable prior to any procedure. Due to the nature of the surgeries being more often focused on primary or secondary sexual organs (e.g., breasts, genitals, reproductive organs), it is not uncommon for people with histories of trauma, and particularly sexual abuse or assault, to experience exacerbations in PTSD symptoms in response to the processes involved in surgery and postsurgical recovery. Assessment of trauma histories and subsequent mental health symptoms is essential. Preparation for surgery can include a discussion of supports to maintain stability of these conditions throughout the entire surgical and recovery period.

In the case of surgeries, support systems and after-care options are a primary focus in preparation and referral. Mental health professionals may be able to refer clients to peer groups and online support groups of individuals considering similar procedures where clients can discuss the experiences with others who have undergone similar surgeries, sometimes with the same surgeons. Housing status and co-habiting friends or family members are important in surgical after-care plans and to assure a safe and relatively clean environment in which to heal. Many surgeries are multi-stage procedures and understanding the timelines (can be up to two years, or more if complications arise) for recovery is essential. Because recovery supports are not always ideal, the mental health provider should assist the client in improving supports and weighing additional options for financing surgery and recovery.

Evaluating how a particular surgery fits into a person's desired transition goals and self-expression is essential. The provider can assist in evaluating the potential impact on life and functioning. For instance, it is not uncommon for non-binary individuals assigned female at birth, and who do not identify as men, to seek chest reconstructive surgery to assist in achieving body comfort and a more androgynous physical appearance. Though less common, it is not unusual for non-binary individuals, assigned male at birth, but who do not identify as women, to seek orchiectomy and for a few who have an *agender* identity, to seek a complete nullification surgery with removal of all external genitalia with no reconstruction. Each person will have a different view of what may relieve their dysphoria. The mental health professional's role is to help the person explore and evaluate the options available as well as the probable social, psychological, and physical outcomes, with the aim of maximizing knowledge and coping skills to undergo the process with resilience.

Preparations and costs of procedures vary, and evaluation of readiness needs to fit the surgery and projected recovery stages and possible complications. Chest reconstructive surgery for transgender masculine individuals, for example, is a relatively easy surgery to undergo and to recover from. It is often done on an outpatient basis and with limited impairment of functioning for a short duration of about 90 days. With some pre-planning, a person can recover well on their own from this procedure. This is much easier to plan for and recover from than genital reconstructive surgery that may require multiple invasive procedures spaced at least 3–6 months apart and possibly demanding significant time off from work. Typically following these surgeries, the client will require assistance with basic self-care and wound management at least during the earliest days postsurgically. A client could be considered well enough prepared for surgery by demonstrating an adequate understanding of the risks and outcomes, including possible complications, of the procedure they seek. The client should have a clear and reasonable plan for the surgery's expected and possible unexpected costs including medications for pain and infection control. In addition, the client should plan for supports and any needed adaptations of their living environment for recovery needs and limitations to mobility or functioning. Finally, the client's medical concerns and mental health issues should be stable and well controlled.

Aging Issues

As transgender people become more visible, there are increasing services and supports available. For instance, there is increasing inclusion of coverage for gender affirming treatments under many private and public insurance plans in the U.S, and the number of individuals seeking treatment is increasing under this expanded access to care. This is particularly seen in older transgender populations who have historically had very limited access to gender affirming treatments. Access to care remains a critical issue within the U.S., nonetheless, and it is common for transgender people to avoid care altogether or not be able to afford care (James et al., 2016).

Outside the U.S., coverage and provision of gender affirming medical treatments also varies. In Canada, England, the Netherlands, and many areas in Europe, transgender care is often covered through national health care plans and unified treatment protocols, though this does not always assure provider competence or even availability of treatments in any particular region to which the individual has access (Ellis, Bailey, & McNeil, 2015). National protocols often have limited flexibility for individuals to access medical transition care who do not identify on a gender binary (Ellis, Bailey, & McNeil, 2015). In some cultures, medical reassignment may be provided by the government, however, it may be used as a way to address proscriptions against homosexuality (e.g., in Iran) and may not be the desired treatment of the individual so much as a way to avoid death (Najmabadi, 2008; 2014). Additionally, outside Westernized cultures, transgender men are largely, or entirely, unheard of (Itthipongmaetee, 2016).As of this writing, coverage for transgender elders and the most marginalized whose care is covered in the U.S. under Medicaid or Medicare plans remains at the discretion of claims reviewers with rare authorizations for treatment even when there are compelling arguments for medical necessity.

In many cultures, transgender elders are at higher risks of poor mental and medical health, disability, and effects of stress than either sexual minorities or the general population (Fredriksen-Goldsen et al., 2013; Koon Teh, 2001). A person's age and age-related health issues may limit the options a person may choose for gender affirmation (Siverskog, 2015) because their age makes them more prone to adverse side effects of treatments. Health concerns and medical conditions may prohibit or greatly limit hormone and surgical treatments in an aged transgender population (Gooren & Lips, 2014). Working collaboratively with a medical provider to support gender affirmation treatments is critical. There may be increased negative effects of stigma and victimization on individuals, necessitating increased advocacy and education on the part of the interdisciplinary team of providers (Fredriksen-Goldsen et al., 2013; Witten, 2014a). Depending on their age, the person may have suppressed their gender expressions or identity for some time (Fabbre, 2014). There may be increased potential losses and pressures from families, spouses, children, and grandchildren to consider when working with an elder transgender individual. There may be increased experiences of violence and elder abuses (Cook-Daniels & munson, 2010) that affect these individuals and their willingness to seek needed care or supports, and there may be a general lack of knowledge about transgender issues and options for self-expression (Siverskog, 2014).

It is common to encounter elder transgender individuals who are unprepared for end-of-life issues and who have significant fears about aging in their natal gender or having their transgender identity discovered when they need assistance with daily living (Witten, 2014b). Common fears include the inability to find welcoming elder care facilities, fears of abuse from caregivers including withholding of hormones, fear of dying alone, and preparations to die by suicide before becoming infirm or dependent (Witten, 2014b). Circumstances and fears may lead some transgender elders to de-transition—or return to their sex assigned at birth—in order to gain access to needed services and supports or to regain family and friends (Koon Teh, 2001; Witten, 2014b). Others may request support for a modified or partial gender transition and expression that allows them to maintain supports and stability in their communities or religious values and rituals (Koon Teh, 2001). These and other issues are illustrated in the case vignettes below.

Case Examples

1. Robert/Barbara is a 68-year-old, white transgender woman. She is a widower with adult children who live elsewhere. She lives 90% of the time as Robert and wishes to have no one know about her gender identity. Barbara wears women's clothes at home in the evenings and weekends. When dressed in feminine clothing Barbara experiences the sense that she is truly herself. She does not want to have genital surgeries. She requests hormone treatments to "grow nice breasts" and reports she wants to present herself as female only on vacations away from home. Barbara is also interested in discussing the option of surgical breast augmentation, which would allow for determination of preferred size in advance and without the risks of feminizing hormones, given her age. However, she also wants to explore her ambivalence and fears of being outed and the effect on her community, church, or home if she lives full time as Barbara. Barbara will benefit from exploring the benefits and limitations of surgical versus non-surgical body modifications. While breast implants would allow her to have a permanent female form with or without hormone treatments, breast forms worn under her clothing might allow her more flexibility and perhaps some safety when she needs to shift presentation from Barbara to Robert. She can remove the forms in a way implants cannot be removed.

   Barbara will benefit from exploring situations such as medical visits for routine and potential emergency care and plan how she may need to manage and plan for voluntary and involuntary disclosure of her female gender identity. Barbara wants to maintain her lifelong positive relationship with her hometown community without changing who they expect her to be (e.g., Robert). She plans to continue living as Robert inside her small town and taking extended trips outside town where she can live for longer periods of time as Barbara. She wants to explore the possibility of living part of the year in a warmer climate as Barbara while spending warmer seasons at home in her historic public identity as Robert. She will need support to explore the challenges and possibilities of increasing her investment in living a dual-gendered life and the potential impact on her as she ages, including exploring probable future needs for assistance in tasks of daily living and how her partially hidden life may affect care options and personal safety. Barbara also wants support to make plans for her children discovering her transgender identity after she dies and she wants to have support to pre-plan and pay for her funeral and grave marker so it reflects her identity.
2. Alex is a 24-year-old who identifies as a "non-binary, sex-positive queer," and primarily socializes with and has romantic partners who are feminine or female. They use gender pronouns they/them/their or just their name Alex, and present as androgynous. Alex is morbidly obese and alternates using men's or women's public restrooms based largely on how they

perceive others' reactions to them and their perceived safety when approaching a restroom.

Alex wants support to manage their anger about public and personal conflicts with strangers who are often hostile when they cannot fit Alex into a gender category and with friends and partners who often misgender or force-fit Alex into their own descriptions and expectations. Alex wants to develop better skills of self-advocacy and assertiveness and is also internally conflicted about exploring hormone therapy as a possibility to more "easily" resolve some of their externally generated stressors due to others being confused by Alex's presentation, thereby reducing the experiences of public and interpersonal conflicts by appearing more unambiguously binary. Alex wants to explore in therapy whether their interest in hormone treatment may be based on a desire to reduce interpersonal conflicts or if it indicates developing changes in their sense of their gender identity. Alex's experience of their body and identity typically do not fit into the roles and expectations typical for either men or women. Alex would ideally like to be able to express gender in a fluid and flexible way and without the need to alter anything about themselves physically to gain public or social approval, but fears this may not be possible without continued personal and social conflicts.

3. Pat is a 36-year-old genderqueer identified person. Pat is partnered with a cisgender woman who identifies as lesbian. Pat is seeking masculinizing chest reconstructive surgery and has no interest in hormone treatments. Pat appears and presents as fairly masculine and identifies as female, using feminine pronouns. She uses men's bathrooms to reduce aggression towards her in public. She is ambivalent about the impact the surgery and her increased masculine appearance will have on her relationship but has marginal interest in exploring this concern in therapy. Pat has money saved and presents a reasonable plan for surgery costs and recovery. She wants help to locate a surgeon who will work with her and acknowledge her feminine identity and simultaneous desire for a masculine chest, and who will provide a good aesthetic and sensate chest outcome without judging her identity.
4. Suzanne is an 18-year-old transgender woman who wants to have genital confirmation surgery during a gap year before college. She lives at home with her parents who are minimally supportive though not rejecting, and she primarily has online friends. She started feminizing hormone treatments two years ago, and has adequate breast development. She has difficulty managing her depression at times and feels this is due to her significant dysphoria related to her body discomfort. She believes genital reconstruction will provide her relief and self-confidence she is lacking now. She wants to explore how she might disclose her transgender history when dating and wants to learn more about possible voice altering surgeries or therapy.

Take Home Points

- Gender identity development and expression are not exclusively binary and can be fluid across the lifespan.
- No two pathways to gender affirmation and expression look the same. Identify the client's goals. Allow the client to lead, while you provide close backup and support with advocacy, referrals, collaboration, and education as needed. Create space for clients' pathways to adjust and change. Sometimes the pathway to gender affirmation is more trail-blazing than following a well-documented roadmap.
- Not all gender diversity, variance, or non-conformity is dysphoria. Assess for dysphoria and separate it from co-occurring mental health issues. Understand and recommend ways to manage either or both and be flexible in assessing which treatment focus is considered paramount.
- Explore and understand intersecting identities and how they impact possible gender affirmation pathways. Understand the cultural, religious and spiritual beliefs or practices, economic status, educational level, racial and ethnic identities, disabilities, and other significant influences on a person and how these interact with the pathways chosen or possible.

Recommended Readings

Jacobs, L. A., Rachlin, K., Erickson-Schroth, L., & Janssen, A. (2014). Gender dysphoria and co-occurring autism spectrum disorders: Review, case examples, and treatment considerations. *LGBT Health, 1*(4), 277–282.

Singh, A. A., and dickey, l. m. (Eds.). (2017). *Affirmative counseling and psychological practice with transgender and gender-nonconforming clients.* Washington, DC: American Psychological Association.

Wylie, K., Barrett, J., Besser, M., Bouman, W. P., Bridgman, M., Clayton, A., … Rathbone, M. (2014). Good practice guidelines for the assessment and treatment of adults with gender dysphoria. *Sexual and Relationship Therapy, 29*(2), 154–214.

References

American Psychological Association. (2015). Guidelines for psychological practice with transgender and gender nonconforming people. *American Psychologist, 70*(9), 832–864. Retrieved from https://www.apa.org/practice/guidelines/transgender.pdf

Beek, T. F., Kreukels, B. P. C., Cohen-Kettenis, P. T., & Steensma, T. D. (2015). Partial treatment requests and underlying motives of applicants for gender affirming interventions. *The Journal of Sexual Medicine, 12*(11), 2201–2205.

Bhasin, S., Safer, J., & Tangpricha, V. (2009). Endocrine treatment of transsexual persons: A patient's guide. Retrieved from www.hormone.org/-/media/hormone/files/patient-guides/mens-health/pgtreatmenttranssexual_2014.pdf

Bockting, W. O., Knudson, G., & Goldberg, J. M. (2007). Counseling and mental health care for transgender adults and loved ones. *International Journal of Transgenderism, 9*(3/4), 35–82.

Boroughs, M. S., Bedoya, C. A., O'Cleirigh, C., & Safren, S. A. (2015). Toward defining, measuring, and evaluating LGBT cultural competence for psychologists. *Clinical Psychology: Science and Practice*, *22*(2), 151–171.

Burnes, T. R., Singh, A. A., Harper, A. J., Harper, B., Maxon-Kann, W., Moundas, S., … Hosea, J. (2010). American Counseling Association *Competencies for counseling with transgender clients*. *Journal of LGBT Issues in Counseling*, *4*(3–4), 135–159. Retrieved from www.tandfonline.com/doi/pdf/10.1080/15538605.2010.524839?needAccess=true

Centers for Disease Control and Prevention. (2017). *Sexual violence: Data sources*. Retrieved from https://www.cdc.gov/violenceprevention/sexualviolence/datasources.html

Chang, S. C., Singh, A. A., & Rossman, K. (2017). Gender and sexual orientation diversity within the TGNC community. In A. A. Singh & l. m. dickey (Eds.), *Affirmative counseling and psychological practice with transgender and gender nonconforming clients* (pp. 19–40). Washington, D.C.: American Psychological Association.

Cook-Daniels, L., & munson, m. (2010). Sexual violence, elder abuse, and sexuality of transgender adults, age 50+: Results of three surveys. *Journal of GLBT Family Studies*, *6*(2), 142–177.

Crossley, S. (2015). Come out, come out, wherever you are: A content analysis of homeless transgender youth in social service literature. *PSU McNair Scholars Online Journal*, *9*(1), Article 4. Retrieved from http://pdxscholar.library.pdx.edu/cgi/viewcontent.cgi?article=1147&context=mcnair

Drescher, J. (2014). Controversies in gender diagnoses. *LGBT Health*, *1*(1), 10–14.

Ellis, S. J., Bailey, L., & McNeil, J. (2015). Trans people's experiences of mental health and gender identity services: A UK study. *Journal of Gay & Lesbian Mental Health*, *19*(1), 4–20.

Enke, F. A. (2016). Stick figures and little bits: Toward a nonbinary pedagogy. In Y. Martínez-San Miguel & S. Tobias (Eds.), *Trans studies: the challenge to hetero/homo normativities* (pp. 215–229). New Brunswick, NJ: Rutgers University Press.

European Union Agency for Fundamental Rights. (2014). *Being trans in the EU - Comparative analysis of the EU LGBT survey data*. European Union Agency for Fundamental Rights (p. 132). Luxembourg. Retrieved from http://fra.europa.eu/en/publication/2014/being-trans-eu-comparative-analysis-eu-lgbt-survey-data

Fabbre, V. D. (2014). Gender transitions in later life: The significance of time in queer aging. *Journal of Gerontological Social Work*, *57*(2–4), 161–175.

Factor, R., & Rothblum, E. (2008). Exploring gender identity and community among three groups of transgender individuals in the United States: MTFs, FTMs, and genderqueers. *Health Sociology Review*, *17*(3), 235–253.

Fredriksen-Goldsen, K. I., Cook-Daniels, L., Kim, H.-J., Erosheva, E. A., Emlet, C. A., Hoy-Ellis, C. P., … Muraco, A. (2013). Physical and mental health of transgender older adults: An at-risk and underserved population. *The Gerontologist*, *54*(3), 488–500.

Gooren, L., & Lips, P. (2014). Conjectures concerning cross-sex hormone treatment of aging transsexual persons. *The Journal of Sexual Medicine*, *11*(8), 2012–2019.

Iantaffi, A., & Bockting, W. O. (2011). Views from both sides of the bridge? Gender, sexual legitimacy and transgender people's experiences of relationships. *Culture, Health & Sexuality*, *13*(3), 355–370.

Itthipongmaetee, C. (June 25, 2016). Transforming transgender health treatment. *Haaretz Daily Newspaper*. Retrieved from www.haaretz.com/world-news/asia-and-australia/1.726938

James, S. E., Herman, J. L., Rankin, S., Keisling, M., Mottet, L., & Anafi, M. (2016). *The Report of the 2015 U.S. Transgender Survey.* Washington, DC: National Center for Transgender Equality. Retrieved from www.transequality.org/sites/default/files/docs/usts/USTS%20Full%20Report%20-%20FINAL%201.6.17.pdf

Koon Teh, Y. (2001). Mak nyahs (male transsexuals) in Malaysia: The influence of culture and religion on their identity. *International Journal of Transgenderism, 5*(3). Retrieved from https://justiceforsisters.files.wordpress.com/2012/08/mak-nyahs-male-transsexuals-in-malaysia.pdf

Lev, A. (2009). The ten tasks of the mental health provider: Recommendations for revision of the World Professional Association for Transgender Health's *Standards of Care. International Journal of Transgenderism, 11*(2), 74–99.

Lombardi, E. L., & van Servellen, G. (2000). Building culturally sensitive substance use prevention and treatment programs for transgendered populations. *Journal of Substance Abuse Treatment, 19*(3), 291–296.

McLemore, K. A. (2015). Experiences with misgendering: identity misclassification of transgender spectrum individuals. *Self & Identity, 14*(1), 51–74.

Meyerowitz, J. J. (2002). *How sex changed: A history of transsexuality in the United States.* Cambridge, MA: Harvard University Press.

Mizock, L., & Fleming, M. Z. (2011). Transgender and gender variant populations with mental illness: Implications for clinical care. *Professional Psychology: Research and Practice, 42*(2), 208–213.

Mizock, L., & Mueser, K. T. (2014). Employment, mental health, internalized stigma, and coping with transphobia among transgender individuals. *Psychology of Sexual Orientation and Gender Diversity, 1*(2), 146–158.

Murad, M. H., Elamin, M. B., Garcia, M. Z., Mullan, R. J., Murad, A., Erwin, P. J., & Montori, V. M. (2010). Hormonal therapy and sex reassignment: A systematic review and meta-analysis of quality of life and psychosocial outcomes. *Clinical Endocrinology, 72*(2), 214–231.

Najmabadi, A. (2008). Transing and transpassing across sex-gender walls in Iran. *Women's Studies Quarterly, 36*(3/4), 23–42.

Najmabadi, A. (2014). *Professing selves: Transsexuality and same-sex desire in contemporary Iran.* Durham, NC: Duke University Press.

Porter, K. E., Ronneberg, C. R., & Witten, T. M. (2013). Religious affiliation and successful aging among transgender older adults: Findings from the Trans MetLife Survey. *Journal of Religion, Spirituality & Aging, 25*(2), 112–138.

Reisner, S. L., White, J. M., Dunham, E. E., Heflin, K., Begenyi, J., Cahill, S., & Project Voice Team. (2014). *Discrimination and health in Massachusetts: A statewide survey of transgender and gender nonconforming adults* (Project VOICE Policy Report) (pp. 1–41). Boston, MA: The Fenway Institute. Retrieved from http://fenwayfocus.org/wp-content/uploads/2014/07/The-Fenway-Institute-MTPC-Project-VOICE-Report-July-2014.pdf

Rettew, D. C. (2012). Apples to committee consensus: The challenge of gender identity classification. *Journal of Homosexuality, 59*(3), 450–459.

Rothman, E. F., Exner, D., & Baughman, A. (2011). The prevalence of sexual assault against people who identify as Gay, Lesbian or Bisexual in the United States: A systematic review. *Trauma, Violence & Abuse, 12*(2), 55–66.

Singh, A. A., & Burnes, T. R. (2010). Shifting the counselor role from gatekeeping to advocacy: Ten strategies for using the *Competencies for Counseling with Transgender Clients* for individual and social change. *Journal of LGBT Issues in Counseling, 4*(3–4), 241–255.

Siverskog, A. (2014). "They just don't have a clue": Transgender aging and implications for social work. *Journal of Gerontological Social Work, 57*(2–4), 386–406.
Siverskog, A. (2015). Ageing bodies that matter: Age, gender and embodiment in older transgender people's life stories. *NORA - Nordic Journal of Feminist and Gender Research, 23*(1), 4–19.
Sperber, J., Landers, S., & Lawrence, S. (2005). Access to health care for transgendered persons: Results of a needs assessment in Boston. *International Journal of Transgenderism, 8*(2-3), 75–91.
White Hughto, J. M., & Reisner, S. L. (2016). A systematic review of the effects of hormone therapy on psychological functioning and quality of life in transgender individuals. *Transgender Health, 1*(1), 21–31.
Witten, T. M. (2014a). It's not all darkness: Robustness, resilience, and successful transgender aging. *LGBT Health, 1*(1), 24–33.
Witten, T. M. (2014b). End of life, chronic illness, and trans-identities. *Journal of Social Work in End-of-Life & Palliative Care, 10*(1), 34–58.
World Professional Association for Transgender Health. (2011). *Standards of care for transsexual, transgender, and gender nonconforming people, Version* 7 (7th ed.). Retrieved from https://s3.amazonaws.com/amo_hub_content/Association140/files/Standards%20of%20Care%20V7%20-%202011%20WPATH%20(2)(1).pdf
World Health Organization. (2017). *Violence and injury prevention*. Retrieved from www.who.int/violence_injury_prevention/violence/world_report/factsheets/en/
Wylie, K., Barrett, J., Besser, M., Bouman, W. P., Bridgman, M., Clayton, A., ... Rathbone, M. (2014). Good practice guidelines for the assessment and treatment of adults with gender dysphoria. *Sexual and Relationship Therapy, 29*(2), 154–214.

6 Preparing Clients for Hormone Therapy

Anthony F. Firek, MS, MD
Ranya Sawan-Garcia, PharmD

The views expressed in this material are those of the authors and do not reflect the official policy or position of the Department of Veterans Affairs or the U.S. Government.

A major objective for most transgender individuals is to achieve the physical characteristics that define their chosen gender. The process to achieve gender affirmation requires that the physical features of their natal sex are diminished and the desired gender features are promoted through the use of specific medications (Bockting et al., 2016). These medications include hormones that are used in a process termed hormone therapy (HT) and are used in combination to achieve the client's transition objectives (Hembree et al., 2009; Wilczynski & Emanuele, 2014; World Professional Association for Transgender Health [WPATH], 2011). Mental health providers should be familiar with the various medications, their realistic effects, and potential adverse events to better support a collaborative relationship with the transgender client and the medical providers in delivery of care. This chapter will provide a guide to understanding the use of these medications.

The effects of many of the medications used in HT are to lower the blood levels of natal sex hormones and decrease their effects within the tissues and organs of the body. In addition, providing cross-sex hormones will directly increase these hormones, resulting in masculinizing or feminizing of the body. This combination approach to medical therapy provides the maximum change in physical appearance for a transgender client. The ultimate goal of HT is to cause changes in gender appearance and bring congruence to an individual's internal experience of gender and external expression of gender while minimizing the risk for adverse medical events. Even though we describe feminizing and masculinizing protocols below, these medications can also be used in non-binary identified clients (for more information about individualizing transition plans see Chapter 5), with the medications used in a manner that is consistent with the individualized treatment plan (e.g., presentation that is more androgynous). The mental health professional plays an essential and key role in this process, not as a gatekeeper, but rather to facilitate success through determining the appropriate diagnosis (i.e., Gender Dysphoria within the Diagnostic and Statistical Manual of Mental Disorders,

5th Edition or Gender Identity Disorder within the International Classification of Diseases, 10th Revision) and discover additional concomitant psychological conditions that may benefit from intervention (American Psychological Association, 2015; Johnson, Shipherd, & Walton, 2016). Mental health providers can also assist in assuring that clients have realistic expectations about the potential effects of hormones. To fully understand the realistic effects and limitations of HT several conversations are usually needed, especially early in therapy as it often takes months to years for full effects to be realized. In addition, determination of the client's realistic understanding of the expected benefits and risks and ability to comply and adhere to a long-term medication program is essential. The interdisciplinary relationship with the medical prescriber is important as this professional support system can assist the client in achieving maximal realistic outcomes (Esteva de Antonio, Gómez-Gil, & GIDSEEN Group, 2013).

The effects of hormones are highly individual, but generally are marked by a receding of natal sex characteristics followed by the development of the sought physical changes (Klaver, Dekker, de Mutsert, Twisk, & den Heijer, 2016). This fact must be emphasized to the transgender client from the initial contact to lessen disappointment based on unrealistic expectations and to reinforce more realistic therapeutic objectives. The physical and mental changes that occur with HT may have profound effects on the client's psycho-social and family dynamics. Transgender people experience a high prevalence of depression, anxiety, and suicidal ideation relative to the general population (Heylens et al., 2014; McCann & Sharek, 2016; Winter et al., 2016). While it is typical that transgender clients experience psychological benefit from HT, due to a lessening of Gender Dysphoria, the changes that occur during HT may also uncover or exacerbate underlying mental health problems.

The medical indication to provide HT is to decrease the significant psychological distress related to the incongruence between the client's sex assigned at birth and actual sense of their gender that meets criteria for a diagnosis of Gender Dysphoria (Hembree et al., 2009). Despite the greater availability of HT to treat Gender Dysphoria, effective psychotherapy for identity consolidation and gender affirming surgery, transgender people may continue to experience higher risks for suicide, drug abuse, HIV infection, homelessness, lower income, and incarceration (Blosnich et al., 2013; Brown & Jones, 2016; Reisner et al., 2016). Many transgender individuals may continue to need involvement with mental health services after medical or surgical interventions for co-occurring conditions (see Chapter 3 for additional information). For more detail about complex presentations see also Chapters 7 and 8.

A key medical therapeutic concept is that HT is not a "one size fits all" intervention. The realistic and expected goals of each transgender client balanced by their individual medical risks are explored and developed into a planned therapeutic program. The key starting point begins with both the mental health and medical provider who are experienced in transgender care making the determination as to eligibility and then readiness for HT (Esteva de Antonio, Gómez-Gil & GIDSEEN Group, 2013; Gardner & Safer, 2013; Wilczynski & Emanuele, 2014). It is important to emphasize to the transgender client that this process is not a barrier to care but rather a way to provide individualized care that will be both effective and safe. The responsibility lays with the mental health provider to assure that the eligibility determination (i.e., a Gender Dysphoria or Gender Identity diagnosis) be viewed as an opportunity to assist the client in reaching their goals. Often this is framed to the client as making sure that their goals are maximized though interdisciplinary team involvement. Elucidation of the client's short- and long-term objectives is essential, along with the realization that objectives may change over the course of medical therapy. The use of HT medications is generally provided in a step-wise fashion to assure tolerability and assess compliance. However, this approach is not mandated and may be modified based on the client's objectives and risks.

Understanding the Effects of Hormone Therapy

While the goal of HT is to lessen distress associated with Gender Dysphoria, some transgender clients may not experience significant dysphoria but are still seeking expert medical guidance on how to achieve their desired gender characteristics. The inability to find help and achieve their desired gender characteristics can over time result in significant distress and would be an indication for HT. Simply asking how an individual would cope without access to HT often validates their underlying concerns.

There are no current United States (U.S.) Food and Drug Administration (FDA) approved medications for use in a HT program and as such these medications are considered "off-label" for this indication. This does not restrict the use of HT as long as there is a proper diagnosis and the client is fully informed of the rational outcomes and potential adverse effects and provides their consent for therapy. Formal written consent, however, is not required to initiate or use HT.

There are currently no clinical trials to help medical providers with objective dose response effects for HT in transgender people. Use is based on expert opinion and experience mainly provided by clinics worldwide with experience in transgender care and guidelines developed by specialty organizations with expertise such as the Endocrine Society and WPATH (Gooren, 2014; Hembree et al., 2009; WPATH, 2011; Wylie et al., 2016).

The success of HT is based on the fact that exposing someone to the hormone that is mainly expressed in the other sex will result in the development of physical changes characteristic of that sex to a varying degree. A natural example is the rare conditions referred to as disorders of sex development (DSD) that previously were called intersex conditions (Byne, 2006; Houk & Lee, 2012). These conditions are often associated with increased sex hormones of the non-natal sex resulting in secondary characteristics that differ from their genetic sex. This is an important issue in transgender care as transgender people may claim a DSD diagnosis to explain their gender identity and desire for masculinizing or feminizing therapy. Transgender people sometimes claim a DSD identity, as they may feel that a medical diagnosis is preferable to a psychological one. For the mental health provider, there is no urgent need to dissuade a client from describing their experience in this way as you can tailor your interventions to this conceptualization until DSD has been ruled out. From a medical perspective, it is important for the provider to have experience with these conditions as diagnosing DSD may require additional testing and then specific therapy. Most transgender people do not have a DSD and can proceed to appropriate HT.

Feminizing Hormone Therapy

The dual objectives in providing HT for transgender women is to promote feminization using a combination of medications to both decrease the levels and effects of testosterone and promote feminization, with an additional goal to maximize safety. In general HT for transgender women is provided to achieve the objectives in a two-stage process beginning with the medications that will lessen the masculine characteristics and then promotion of feminization with the use of estradiol. This approach allows the transgender woman the opportunity to engage in the transition focusing on these objectives sequentially and safely. This approach can help reinforce the client's understanding of HT benefits and risks. It allows the transgender woman and the therapist to gauge the effects of each stage, evaluate and reinforce compliance and to determine any adverse effects of individual medications. A summary of the various medications available for HT for transgender women is shown in Table 6.1 below.

Table 6.1 Medications that are available for feminizing hormone therapy

Medication	*Use*	*Recommended*	*Reason*	*Comments*
Estradiol (17-β)	Feminization	Yes	Improved safety and identical to natural estrogen.	Transdermal preferred with Sublingual an option. Injections not recommended.
Premarin	Feminization	No	Increased risk. Cannot monitor levels.	Commonly used in clinical practice.
Oral contraceptives (Ethinyl estradiol)	Feminization	No	Increased risk. Cannot monitor levels.	

(continued)

Table 6.1. Medications that are available for feminizing hormone therapy *(continued)*

Medication	*Use*	*Recommended*	*Reason*	*Comments*
Progesterone	Feminization. Breast enhancement	No	No proven benefit. Increased risk in combination with estradiol.	May use on a temporary basis to lower testosterone.
Spironolactone	Decreases masculinization	Yes	Safe and moderately effective.	Must monitor kidney function and potassium.
Finasteride	Decreases masculinization	Yes	Safe.	Uncertain if effective.
Flutamide	Decreases masculinization	No	Blocks testosterone. Unsafe for the liver.	
GnRH	Decreases masculinization	Yes, in selected patients	Very effective at lowering testosterone.	Injections and should be limited to 3 years or less.

The potential changes that occur with feminization are shown in Table 6.2. This table serves as a way to discuss and objectively measure goals with the transgender client undergoing HT. However, as previously mentioned, both the time to onset and maximum feminization is highly variable for each person. Pre-existing male characteristics often make the transition to a feminized appearance difficult and unsatisfactory for the transgender woman.

Table 6.2 Summary of expected feminizing changes with hormone therapy

Changes	*Onset*	*Maximum effect*
Redistribution of body fat	3–6 months	2–3 years
Decrease in muscle mass and strength	3–6 months	1–2 years
Softening of skin/decreased oiliness	3–6 months	Unknown
Decreased libido	1–3 months	3–6 months
Decreased spontaneous erections	1–3 months	3–6 months
Male sexual dysfunction	Variable	Variable
Breast growth	3–6 months	2–3 years
Decreased testicular volume	3–6 months	2–3 years
Decrease sperm production	Unknown	> 3 years
Decreased terminal hair growth	6–12 months	> 3 years
Scalp hair	No regrowth	May have some regrowth > 3 years
Voice changes	None	May have some change > 3 years

Expected effects of feminizing hormone therapy are increased breast size, decreased facial hair, softening of skin and facial features, decreased skin oiliness, redistribution of body fat towards the buttocks, hips, and thighs supporting a feminine shape/appearance, and decreased muscle mass most notably in the torso area. These clinical objectives of body changes are believed to occur when the transgender woman can achieve a blood level of estradiol that is approximate to those in natal females. Medical therapists will use a level of ~ 200 pg/ml as the maximum estradiol level based on minimizing risk for estradiol use. The concomitant objective is to decrease the blood testosterone to the natal female range of < 55 ng/dl (Hembree et al., 2009). The goal of any specific HT regimen is therefore not to exceed this level of estradiol for safety and to suppress testosterone. It should be noted that these therapeutic targets are based on expert opinion (Hembree et al., 2009; WPATH, 2011) and not on randomized clinical trials. Much of the "art" of transgender medicine is finding the specific regimen that will achieve these therapy goals and is also acceptable to the client.

There are limitations to feminization therapy that should be carefully spelled-out prior to the initiation of HT to address unrealistic expectations. For example, the breast enlargement associated with HT may not be sufficient for some clients (maximum growth observed is a B-size cup) resulting in their seeking additional enhancement interventions such as implants. It should be noted that WPATH (2011) recommends that clients be on feminizing hormones for a year to allow maximal breast development prior to undergoing breast augmentation surgery. Body and facial hair growth may slow and become thinner, but overall hair growth suppression, particularly beard growth, is usually not adequate with hormone therapy alone. Individuals often choose to pursue adjunctive cosmetic services or products to remove facial hair (see Chapter 10 for additional information about adjunctive interventions). Feminization therapy also does not lessen the prominence of the laryngeal cartilage, commonly called the Adam's apple, nor does it affect vocal pitch. The enlarged cartilage can be reduced by a surgical shave procedure. Vocal characteristics including pitch, inflection, and manner of speech can be improved through vocal coaching and speech therapy (McNeill, 2006). Specialists in this area include speech language pathologists, speech therapists, and speech-voice clinicians. Offering this service to the transgender woman is an important value-added benefit to HT. (See Chapter 10 for more information).

One important issue to address is that estradiol can have irreversible effects on sexual and gonadal function, including decreased libido, testicular size, and decreased spontaneous erections. These effects can lead to erectile dysfunction. Use of HT may also cause decreased sperm production leading to irreversible infertility. Both the mental health and medical providers must have frank and open discussions about the loss of libido and sexual functioning, as well as potential infertility, prior to initiation of HT. Fertility concerns and options for sperm preservation are crucial discussion points if the client is interested in having children in the future. This discussion also should include counseling concerning safe sex practices, as transgender women have a higher risk of sexual transmitted diseases, especially HIV infection (De Roo, Tilleman, T'Sjoen, & De Sutter, 2016; Herbst et al., 2008; Neumann, Finlayson, Pitts, & Keatley, 2017).

Medications Used in Feminization

Estradiol

The primary feminizing hormone in a HT regimen for transgender women is estradiol. Estradiol is the hormone produced by the ovaries in natal females. Estradiol will in general promote female secondary sex characteristics and suppress the expression of male secondary sex characteristics both directly in the tissue and by suppressing testosterone secretion. The 17-β estradiol is the recommended estradiol formulation for use in HT as it is thought to have fewer associated risks for medical complications than other types of estrogen (Olié, Canonico, & Scarabin, 2010). Estradiol can be given by mouth, under the tongue (sublingual), applied to the skin in a transdermal patch, or by injection. Compounding pharmacies can also provide custom transdermal creams and gels for use in HT, but these are not validated as consistently effective. The choice of an estradiol product is based in part on the client's concomitant medical conditions and medical risks factors for adverse events. In the U.S., the FDA has found the recommended estradiol preparations to be generally effective in natal women, and the potential adverse effects are generally well known. However, estradiol has not been FDA approved for use in transgender women.

Estrogen in any form, including estradiol, increases the propensity for the blood to form clots within leg, lung, heart blood vessels, and blood vessels within the brain (see Table 6.3). These clotting effects and other effects on blood vessels could lead to heart attack, stroke, or adverse effects on lung function (Gooren, Wierckx, & Giltay, 2014; Wierckx et al., 2013). Therefore, using any estradiol formulation requires the medical provider to determine the risks in the client for a stroke, blood clots, and a heart attack. These risks significantly increase in people who are obese, smokers, and older than 35 years of age. Heart attack and stroke risks include diabetes, elevated cholesterol and blood pressure, and sedentary lifestyle among others. Estradiol can also potentially increase the risk for breast cancer in natal males and must be evaluated over time by family risk, breast exams, and mammograms. Use of other estrogen containing products such as conjugated estrogens (Premarin® Pfizer, Inc.) or oral contraceptives are not recommended as they may increase the risk of adverse events compared to estradiol and provide no therapeutic advantage over estradiol. In addition, conjugated hormone levels cannot be monitored as well as estradiol. Premarin® and oral contraceptives can be readily obtained by clients from non-prescribed sources such as the Internet and less experienced medical providers. Therefore, it is important to advise the client about these concerns.

Table 6.3 Risks associated with feminizing hormone therapy

Risk level (Low, moderate, or high rating)	*Clinical outcome*
High	Venous thromboembolic disease Hypertriglyceridemia Gallstones Elevated liver enzymes Weight gain
High with presence of additional risk factors	Cardiovascular disease
Moderate	Hypertension Elevated prolactin or development of a prolactin secreting tumor
Moderate with additional risks such as obesity, family history, ethnic origin	Type 2 diabetes
Low or inconclusive	Breast cancer

The preferred formulation of estradiol is transdermal estradiol. These products are readily available as skin patches and release estradiol through the skin into the blood vessels. Transdermal estradiol patches are changed weekly and may therefore enhance individual compliance with estradiol use. The release of estradiol through the skin causes the estradiol in large part to bypass the intestine and liver. Both the intestine and liver can change estradiol when taken by mouth to inactive forms and, more importantly, alter the production of various proteins in the blood that increases the risk for blood clotting. Transdermal estradiol minimizes but does not eliminate this risk. Transdermal estradiol is the recommended formulation for individuals with increased risk for blood clots and cardiovascular disease, such as transgender women over the age of 40, smokers, obese, immobilized individuals with uncontrolled risk factors, or those who have a family history of blood clots in the legs or lungs.

Other formulations of estradiol such as the oral formulations are available, including using estradiol under the tongue (sublingual) and tablets that are swallowed. The sublingual formulation is used to lessen the risk of blood clots compared to swallowed estradiol tablets because it is absorbed into the bloodstream largely bypassing the liver.

In healthy ambulating, non-smoking, individuals who are less than 40 years of age, all forms of estradiol— oral, sublingual, or transdermal—are reasonable options for HT. The choice is largely determined by the client's preference after medication counseling.

Injectable estradiol (estradiol valerate) is available in a depot form that can be self-injected weekly into the muscle. Transgender women often request this form of estradiol with the objective of getting as much estrogen into their body as possible. Some medical providers prefer this formulation without evidence of any superior benefits. The injectable form can produce highly variable and extreme levels of estradiol in the blood, placing the transgender woman at risk for adverse events. Injectable estradiol is generally not recommended for routine use (Hembree et al., 2009; WPATH, 2011).

Spironolactone

The medication spironolactone is in general use in clinical medicine as a diuretic (water pill) and to help control blood pressure. It was found early on to increase breast swelling and tenderness in natal males, and this effect was discovered to be related to lower testosterone levels in the blood and blocked testosterone effects in certain organs, particularly the chest. It has been adapted for use in HT to oppose testosterone and is therefore called an "anti-androgen." Spironolactone is used to decrease the masculine features of the transgender woman by blocking testosterone (Prior, Vigna, & Watson, 1989; Rose, Underwood, Newmark, Kisch, & Williams, 1977). Medications like spironolactone are usually given with estradiol to enhance the feminizing effects of estradiol because inhibiting testosterone allows for more effective estradiol effects and potentially lowers the dose of estrogen needed to achieve the desired goals.

Being a diuretic and a medication that can affect blood pressure, the major risks for the use of spironolactone is that it may adversely affect kidney functions and affect the potassium in the blood. Spironolactone can cause potassium to rise to dangerous levels. Consequently, potassium and kidney function are monitored during therapy. Spironolactone can also cause distressing breast tenderness and reduction in sex drive.

Finasteride

This medication decreases the production of the active form of testosterone called 5-alpha dihydrotestosterone (5-DHT). Finasteride is commonly used to treat adult natal males with an enlarged prostate. Use of finasteride in transgender women, therefore, is based on this action in natal males to inhibit the effects of testosterone in tissue. The efficacy and safety of use data in transgender people is largely anecdotal and based on the effects in cisgender men. Finasteride may improve male-pattern baldness, and it also has positive effects on breast development in transgender women. Although generally considered safe, adverse effects include decreased libido, erectile dysfunction, and depression.

Flutamide

Flutamide is known to inhibit the binding of testosterone in various tissues with the potential to decrease the effects of testosterone. It has no effect on testosterone levels (Koulouri & Conway, 2008). Flutamide is sometimes used in transgender women. However, it is toxic to the liver and lacks demonstrated efficacy in feminization and, therefore, is not recommended for use in HT.

Progesterone

Progesterone is a natural hormone produced in natal women at various times during the menstrual cycle and during pregnancy. The chemically derived progesterone—medroxyprogesterone—was a popular therapy in natal women on concomitant estrogen therapy in the past. Subsequent studies such as the Women's Health Initiative have demonstrated that progesterone in combination with estrogens such as Premarin® resulted in increased net harm to women by increasing heart attack and stroke risk and breast cancer (Gurney, Nachtigall, Nachtigall, & Naftolin, 2014).

Other formulations such as micronized progesterone are available, but there is no evidence this preparation improves safety (Mueck, 2012). Medical providers in transgender medicine use progesterone at times to enhance suppression of testosterone with estradiol therapy. Transgender women will often request progesterone as an additional feminizing hormone to enhance the effects of estradiol, particularly for breast development and to promote other less defined feminine qualities. While the lore among the transgender community is that progesterone is necessary to fully feminize, there are no published comparative clinical studies showing that progesterone in any form enhances breast development to any significant degree or is necessary for increasing feminization.

The medications within the class called gonadotropin-releasing hormone (GnRH) agonists such as Luprolide and Goserelin that can be used in both transgender men and women are described below.

Medical Risk Outcomes in Feminizing Hormone Therapy

Most concerns about adverse events caused by feminizing HT are largely based on the known risks of using estradiol therapy in natal women. Tables 6.3 and 6.4 summarize the known risks for estradiol. Therapy using spironolactone has well-defined adverse effects related to blood pressure, kidney function, and electrolytes such as potassium. The concern about concomitant use of progesterone with estradiol also comes from studies in natal women, particularly the Women's Health Initiative as noted previously.

Table 6.4 Medical conditions that can be worsened by estrogen therapy

Very high risk of serious adverse outcome	*Moderate to high risk of adverse outcome*
Blood clots in the legs or lungs (venous thromboembolic disease)	Pituitary tumors secreting prolactin Abnormal liver function Breast cancer Atherosclerotic vascular disease of the heart or brain Onset or worsening of migraine headaches

There is a lack of well-documented longitudinal outcome studies examining adverse outcomes among transgender women using HT. Evidence to date has been based on observational clinic experiences, uncontrolled retrospective surveys, and case studies as discussed below.

A recent study from the Netherlands evaluated mortality in their clinic group of transgender people for up to 18 years (Asscheman et al., 2011). There were no specific adverse outcomes related to HT except in the use of a type of estrogen called ethinyl estradiol. Current but not past users of this form of estrogen demonstrated an increased cardiovascular mortality by three-fold.

The overall total mortality was 51% higher for transgender women compared to the general population, but mainly from suicide, HIV/AIDS, cardiovascular disease, drug abuse, and unknown causes (Asscheman et al., 2011). There was no increase in total cancer mortality, but lung and hematological cancer mortality rates were increased. The transgender group did have a higher smoking rate that may have been the contributing risk to this finding. An increased risk of suicide was also found in a recent study of transgender veterans at Veterans Health Administration (VHA) facilities with a 20 times increased rate of suicidal gestures as compared with veterans in VHA generally (Blosnich et al., 2013). Data also suggested that suicide might occur at a younger overall age among transgender veterans than in the general veteran population (Blosnich, Brown, Wojcio, Jones, & Bossarte, 2014).

A recent review of the literature concluded that HT in transgender adults is considered safe when used by a provider with experience or proper provider supervision (Weinand & Safer, 2015). A review of HT outcomes for transgender individuals found that the major risk for feminizing HT was the development of venous thrombosis events (stroke) and increased triglycerides (Weinand & Safer, 2015). No increase in cancer or mortality could be attributed to HT. These recent findings are consistent with the risks described in WPATH *Standards of Care* (2011).

Aside from the recognized risk for the development of blood clots within veins, studies from Europe have suggested that HT in transgender women carries an increased risk for cerebral and cardiac events, such as myocardial infarction compared to natal women (Wierckx et al., 2013). However, the event rates appear to be consistent with that of natal males and are likely related to other risk factors among transgender women. Thus, it does not appear that HT use in transgender women is a major contributing risk for heart attacks or strokes. However, with pre-existing risks, aggressive risk modification is clearly important.

Other established risks of estrogen therapy include fluid retention and fertility impairment that may be permanent. Hormonally sensitive tumors including prolactinomas, breast cancer, and prostate cancer are potential risks of estrogen therapy, although evidence is limited and causality has not been established. There are reports in the literature of the development of cancers such as breast cancer with use of HT (Gooren, van Trotsenburg, Giltay, & van Diest, 2013). However, other studies have not shown increased risk for breast cancer, at least in U.S. veterans (Brown & Jones 2015). Therefore, it is important to follow established screening protocols for detection of known cancers related to the client's natal sex and for breast cancer in transgender people taking feminizing HT. Lastly, studies have found that HT increases insulin resistance and blood glucose levels and places transgender women at risk for diabetes mellitus (Gooren, Giltay, & Bunck, 2008).

Medications used to lower or block testosterone may adversely affect bone density and may increase the risk for osteoporosis and bone fractures. Prolonged use of HT therapy without estradiol may decrease bone density significantly (Lapauw et al., 2008). Evaluation of bone density by bone densitometry or DEXA (dual-energy x-ray absorptiometry) scanning is prudent for transgender women over 55 years of age, particularly with additional risk factors for osteoporosis. The incidence of osteoporosis-related fractures among transgender women or men is unknown.

Masculinizing Hormone Therapy

The primary goals of masculinizing HT are to induce masculine physical characteristics and reduce natal female characteristics. The goals are achieved by increasing the blood levels of testosterone and lowering the natal levels of estradiol. Physical changes caused by testosterone occur over the course of months to years and are often irreversible. Table 6.5 summarizes the expected changes with therapy. Table 6.6 below summarizes the medications used in HT for transgender men.

Changes expected within the first 6 months of therapy include cessation of menses, which is an anticipated goal of masculinization therapy. Testosterone will cause increased oily skin and acne and redistribution of body fat from hips, thighs, and buttocks to the abdomen, resulting in a more masculine physique. Additional changes with testosterone include clitoral enlargement and vaginal atrophy (Hembree et al., 2009). Testosterone may cause infertility that may be permanent and, therefore, oocyte cryopreservation (freezing

Table 6.5 Summary of masculinizing changes with hormone therapy

Changes	*Onset*	*Maximum*
Skin oiliness and acne	1–6 months	1–2 years
Facial/body hair growth	6–12 months	4–5 years
Scalp hair loss	6–12 months	
Increased muscle mass/strength	6–12 months	2–5 years
Fat re-distribution	1–6 months	2–5 years
Cessation of menses	2–6 months	Continued or resumption of menses requires evaluation
Clitoral enlargement	3–6 months	1–2 years
Vaginal atrophy	3–6 months	1–2 years
Deepening of voice	6–12 months	1–2 years

Table 6.6 Medical conditions that may worsen with testosterone therapy

High risk of serious adverse events	*Moderate to high risk of serious events*
Breast or uterine cancer Increased red blood cell mass (Erythrocytosis-Hematocrit > 50%)	Severe liver dysfunction[a]

Note: [a] Liver function tests that are greater than 3 times the upper limit of normal. This is more common with oral products.

eggs) may need to be discussed. Other changes expected to occur within the first year of HT include increased facial hair growth (mustache and/or beard growth), increased body hair growth (arms, legs, chest, abdomen, and back), deepening of the voice, possible scalp hair loss (male pattern baldness), and increased muscle mass and strength. Scalp hair loss is highly dependent on predisposed genetic factors, such as family history as well as age. Increased muscle mass and strength development varies and are significantly dependent on the amount of exercise and weight training the client pursues to foster this physical trait.

Masculinizing Medications

Testosterone

Various testosterone products are available for administration using transdermal patch or gel, injection, or pill. Testosterone administration in pill form is not recommended due to the significant risk of liver toxicity. Transdermal patch or gel and injection are the preferred choices in a masculinizing HT regimen, although there are no comparative effectiveness studies to date (Irwig, 2017). Injectable depot testosterone products, cypionate or enanthate, are long-acting formulations and can be effectively administered weekly or once every two weeks into the muscle. Testosterone undecanoate is a unique, long-acting testosterone preparation that only requires injection every 10 weeks (Jacobeit, Gooren, & Schulte, 2009). The standard injectable preparations of testosterone are often associated with cyclic fluctuations in hormone levels and may have respective adverse effects on mood, energy, and libido. Transdermal testosterone preparations provide a more consistent release of hormone levels and are available as patch, gel, or solution. Transdermal patches can cause skin irritation, while the testosterone gel and solution pose a risk of secondary transfer; that is, exposure of testosterone to unintended individuals, such as women and children who come into contact with treated skin or unwashed clothing. The decision regarding selection of product should be a personal choice based on advantages and disadvantages of each preparation.

Testosterone is teratogenic and contraindicated during pregnancy. While testosterone can suppress menses in the transgender man, ovulation may still occur. Testosterone therapy is not an effective method of contraception, nor will it prevent sexually transmitted infections. Contraceptive counseling and an effective form of birth control are required for transgender men on testosterone therapy of childbearing age. Safe sex practices should also be discussed with all transgender individuals.

Progesterone

Progesterone preparations do not have properties that affect the development of male secondary sex characteristics and are not typically included in a masculinizing HT regimen. However, progesterone can be used short term to cause cessation of menstrual bleeding, particularly at the start of testosterone HT. Depot medroxyprogesteroneacetate (DMPA—Depo-Provera® and generic formulations) can be given every three months at the start of testosterone therapy and has the added benefit of providing an effective form of contraception if used long term in the sexually active transgender man.

Gonadotropin-releasing hormone (GnRH) agonists

Medications in this class can be used in HT for either transgender women or men and include Goserelin or Luprolide, both of which are available as generics. Administration of a GnRH agonist by injection will cause a suppression of the hormones (gonadotropins) produced in the part of the brain called the pituitary, which regulates testosterone or estradiol. The result is a profound suppression of the respective natal hormones. GnRH agonists are given as monthly or quarterly injections and are highly effective in decreasing levels of testosterone or estradiol. With administration of GnRH agonists, there is a sustained suppression of testosterone or estradiol levels that fall into the range normally seen in surgically castrated natal males or females (Dittrich et al., 2005). Some common (> 10% incidence) adverse effects of GnRH agonist therapy include headaches, peripheral edema, peripheral vasodilation, hot flashes, depression, and emotional labiality. GnRH agonists can cause heart conduction delays that may be serious. While beyond the scope of this chapter, it is worth mentioning that medications in this class are also often used to delay puberty in transgender children in order to give them more time to consolidate their gender identity and develop transition plans before irreversible physical changes take place or are induced.

Medical Risk Outcomes in Masculinizing Hormone Therapy

Testosterone therapy has been used for decades in hypogonadal natal males, and there is a well-defined set of adverse effects and noted risks with its use. The same precautions should be followed when used in transgender men. Tables 6.7 and 6.8 list both the medical conditions and risks that should be evaluated and managed. Recent concern has been raised about the safety of testosterone in natal males for possible increased cardiovascular risk leading to

Table 6.7 Risks associated with masculinizing hormone therapy

Risk level (Low, moderate, or high rating)	*Outcome*
High	Increased red cell mass of the blood—polycythemia Weight gain Acne Androgenic alopecia (male pattern baldness) Sleep apnea
Moderate	Elevated liver enzymes Elevated blood lipids—hyperlipidemia
Moderate risk with the presence of additional risk factors	Destabilization of certain psychiatric disorders Cardiovascular disease Hypertension Type 2 diabetes
Low or inconclusive	Loss of bone density Breast cancer Cervical cancer Ovarian cancer Uterine cancer

Table 6.8 Summary table of masculinizing medications*

Medication	*Use*	*Recommended*	*Reason*	*Comments*
Testosterone	Masculinization	Yes	Most effective	Gel or patch preferred. Injections less optimal due to variable levels. Oral testosterone not recommended.
Progesterone	Menses cessation/ contraception	Yes, temporary to stop menses	Effective	Depot Provera may be used for contraception
GnRH	Decreases feminization or masculinization depending on natal sex	Yes, in selected patients	Very effective at lowering estradiol	Injections and should be limited to 3 years or less

Note: *GnRH agonists can be used for masculinization or feminization

heart attacks and strokes (Oskui et al., 2013). The medical provider should consider possible cardiovascular risks of testosterone use in transgender men. Testosterone therapy is contraindicated for use in individuals with hormone sensitive cancers, such as breast or uterine cancer because these cancers may progress with exposure to testosterone. Testosterone therapy is known to increase the red blood cell mass and may result in increases in the thickness of the blood with increased risk for stroke. Testosterone can adversely affect liver function, and its use is in a transgender man with moderate-to-severe liver dysfunction is not indicated (Fernández-Balsells et al., 2010).

Skin changes and loss of hair are often disturbing but can be managed with topical or systemic agents. Testosterone in particular can increase known vascular risks such as adverse lipid changes, induction or worsening of sleep apnea, and increased blood pressure. Infertility can occur and, as noted earlier, testosterone is not an effective contraceptive, and fetal exposure can be teratogenic. Adverse psychological effects have been associated with testosterone therapy in individuals with pre-existing mental health conditions, including bipolar depression, schizoaffective disorder, and other disorders that may include manic or psychotic symptoms.

The limited number of outcome studies to date have not demonstrated that testosterone therapy increases adverse events or increases mortality in transgender people. There are few studies in this area but the quality of evidence is low (Pope, Kouri & Hudson, 2000).

Special Concern regarding HIV Infection and HT

Transgender women are at particularly high risk for HIV infection. In fact, African American transgender women and other women of color have the highest rate for new HIV infection of all groups of at-risk individuals (Nuttbrock et al., 2009; Operario, Soma, & Underhill, 2008). Transgender sex workers have a particularly high prevalence rate for HIV. Several factors contribute to increased HIV infection rates among transgender women, including higher rates of sexually transmitted infections, decreased access to healthcare with providers who have competency in providing transgender-related care, discrimination in workplaces and housing, and financial constraints which can contribute to sex work appeal.

Transgender individuals on HIV anti-retroviral therapy and concomitant HT may have serious drug–drug interactions and adverse effects that need to be considered. There is a potential reduction in estrogen levels with HIV medication use. This may lead to transgender women decreasing anti-retroviral medication adherence or increasing estrogen administration to overcome any deficit in estradiol levels. For this reason, assessment of medication adherence is critical to ensure suppression of viral load and avoid additional risks associated with excessive estrogen utilization. Certain HIV therapies also may interact with testosterone. This may result in inhibition of liver metabolism with subsequent increases in testosterone levels or inhibition or competitive binding of a key metabolic protein leading to increased levels of anti-retroviral therapy or testosterone. For transgender men who take testosterone, vaginal thinning and atrophy often occur, which can raise the risk of acquiring HIV through the vaginal mucosa during sexual intercourse. The increased risk for HIV and possibly other sexually transmitted diseases requires that a discussion and counseling on safe sex practices be a part of HT.

The Medical and Mental Health Provider Collaboration in HT Management

The medical provider is tasked with providing an effective and safe medication program to the transgender client. Usually an endocrinologist will be the primary medical provider for a transgender client, but other medically qualified providers such as psychiatrists or primary care providers can serve in that capacity. The key issue is experience and expertise in a holistic approach to medical therapy for transgender individuals. Expertise in HT is generally obtained through didactic educational programs, peer mentoring, and practical clinical experience. There are no currently recognized certification programs such as postgraduate medicine fellowships in transgender medicine in the U.S. at this time.

The U.S. Veterans Health Administration (VHA) has instituted a unique and highly innovative nation-wide program using peer-to-peer training and the use of e-consults to provide direct expertise in both mental health and medical recommendations tailored to each unique transgender veteran's treatment plan (Kauth et al., 2015; Shipherd, Kauth, & Matza, 2016).

As noted previously, the mental health professional plays a key and collaborative role in the delivery of HT. Mental health interventions are particularly important for risk factor modification. Most medical practitioners assess risk based on established protocols derived from the non-transgender population, which may not apply to a transgender client. Risk factor identification is followed by risk modification interventions, including education, medications, and possible behavioral modification guided by a mental health provider. Because changes in lifestyle (e.g., smoking cessation) are particularly challenging, mental health providers can be effective in promoting change and reducing health risk.

In short, the three most concerning adverse medical outcomes with HT are the development of blood clots (venous thrombosis), cardio-cerebral vascular disease, and cancer. The medical provider determines a level of absolute and relative risk for these adverse events at the time of HT initiation and in the future and then identifies the critical lifestyle interventions that should be instituted. The mental health professional plays a critical role in reinforcing healthy behaviors and choices, maintaining adherence, and helping the individual maximize coping skills. Specifically, adopting a healthy diet with exercise and reducing or stopping smoking significantly decreases cardiovascular risk.

Evaluation of blood pressure, blood lipid levels, and blood glucose levels are important in advance of starting HT. Evaluating pre-existing medical conditions and the effects of HT is also part of the initial and ongoing task of the medical provider. Adjusting or adding other medications may be necessary prior to and during HT. For example, a transgender woman with hypertension may need to lower her existing regimen when adding spironolactone for its anti-androgen effects because this medication also lowers blood pressure. Identification of risks for blood clots that may develop in the veins is critical and may require adjustment of estradiol or testosterone in transgender women at high risk. A strong recommendation to stop smoking is critical, as this is one of the most important modifiable risks for thrombosis. Behavioral modification techniques with the use of nicotine replacement can be particularly effective (Siu, 2015). The decision to use HT in a transgender person who continues to smoke must be carefully weighed against the risks of complications versus the potential adverse effects of withholding HT from that individual and the likelihood of the client seeking readily available non-prescribed medications (see case examples below).

Conclusion

There is a reassuring lack of published evidence that HT increases the risk for cancer in either transgender men or women above a similar natal gender population. However, discussion with clients about the possible risk of cancer with HT is important, along with recommendations for health screening based on the duration of exposure to HT, age, and other attended risks. Routine health screening for transgender clients must be instituted based on the duration of HT. Despite exposing transgender women to estradiol, there is no compelling evidence of an increase in breast cancer based on the current published literature but other cancers remain unstudied. Lastly, the transgender population has an increased risk for depression, suicide, HIV infection, and substance abuse relative to the general population. A partnership with mental health professionals is essential to providing counseling and intervention that often cannot be delivered by the medical provider.

Case Studies

1. A 31-year-old natal male with a chosen name of Jane presents to her family doctor with a strong commitment to begin HT. She met once with a mental health professional who is unknown to the medical provider and who provided a note stating, "Jane is cleared for hormones." Jane is a heavy smoker and obese with high blood pressure. She has obtained Premarin® from the Internet and uses it intermittently.

   Discussion: This is a common scenario in transgender medicine in which a client presents to their medical provider with either no mental health evaluation or inadequate documentation of an evaluation and having tried self-administered HT medications. Discussion of preferred name and pronoun choice is important at the first interaction. Jane's smoking and obesity place her at increased risk for medical complications, and she has used a form of estrogen that significantly increases her risk for vascular complications. The first step is to immediately counsel Jane on the inherent risks of using any non-prescribed medication and to work diligently on risk modification, particularly smoking cessation. Starting an anti-androgen such as spironolactone or even a GnRH agonist could be initiated even with her continued smoking. Referral to both an experienced mental health provider is warranted and a medical provider experienced in HT.

2. Ed is 29-year-old transgender man who was appropriately diagnosed with Gender Dysphoria under DSM-5 by a mental health professional and has the capacity to make an informed medical decision. Ed has had appropriate counseling on the risks and benefits of testosterone therapy and has started treatment by injecting testosterone every week. However, after three months of testosterone therapy, he complains to his endocrinologist that he does not feel satisfied with the results of the treatment and wants to double the dose of testosterone. Ed also continues to have unprotected receptive sex with his male partner.

   Discussion: Often transgender people are unsatisfied with the physical effects of HT. The immediate request is to increase the dose, without an appreciation for the time it takes for the effects to be apparent. Ed should be counseled to reinforce the fact that effects are variable and more medication will not make him look more masculine and may place him at increased risk for adverse effects of testosterone therapy. Reviewing the expected changes and the time frame for those changes is important. Reviewing his lab testing will reveal if he is self-adjusting his testosterone appropriately. Ed may be at risk for pregnancy as testosterone is not an effective contraceptive. Ed may also be at risk for sexually transmitted infections. Urgent counseling is needed to address these issues. Ideally the medical provider requests a clinic visit with both the client and his partner and the mental health provider and endocrinologist.

3. Sarah is a 75-year-old transgender woman who was recently evaluated by a mental health provider and is eligible for HT. Sarah states she is "ready to blossom" as a woman but has never taken any HT. She has a history of prostate cancer, myocardial infarction, and hepatitis C and lives alone in her own home. Sarah does not want to come out to her family and uses her given name, Tom, and dresses as a male when around her family. In all other situations, Sarah presents as a woman.

   Discussion: Older transgender people who request HT pose unique challenges for both mental health and medical providers. Sarah has many medical risk factors and concurrent medical conditions that raise concerns about initiating HT. She may have highly unrealistic expectations about what physical transformations can take place given her age. She also has chosen to live in two gender scenarios and lacks support from her family and perhaps anticipates hostility if they knew about her gender identity. Work with a mental health professional may help boost her social support and better prepare her for coming out to her family if/when she is ready. Moreover, given her age, discussion is warranted about elder housing options where she could have support throughout her advancing years in case her family rejects her transitioning. Given Sarah's significant medical risks, the HT recommended for her was to use a GnRH agonist alone without estradiol. Continued counseling and support resulted in her acceptance of this approach.

Take Home Points

- Optimal HT is accomplished through the collaboration of care with multiple specialties including gynecology, mental health, primary care, endocrinology, women's health, and pharmacy.
- All transgender clients must be counseled on the benefits, risks, realistic expectations, limitations, and reversible and irreversible effects of HT, as well as fertility options.
- All transgender individuals should be educated on safe sex practices and risks associated with sexually transmitted diseases and infections.

Recommended Readings

Ettner, R. (2013). Care of the elderly transgender patient. *Current Opinion in Endocrinology, Diabetes, and Obesity, 20*(6), 580–584.

Joseph, A., Cliffe, C., Hillyard, M., & Majeed, A. (2017). Gender identity and the management of the transgender patient: A guide for non-specialists. *Journal of the Royal Society of Medicine, 110*(4), 144–152. Doi: 10.1177/0141076817696054

White Hughto, J. M., & Reisner, S. L. (2016). A systematic review of the effects of hormone therapy on psychological functioning and quality of life in transgender individuals. *Transgender Health, 1*(1), 21–31.

References

American Psychological Association. (2015). Guidelines for psychological practice with transgender and gender nonconforming people. *American Psychologist, 70*(9), 832–864. Retrieved from https://www.apa.org/practice/guidelines/transgender.pdf

Asscheman, H., Giltay, E. J., Megens, J. A., de Ronde, W. P., van Trotsenburg, M. A., & Gooren, L. J. (2011). A long-term follow-up study of mortality in transsexuals receiving treatment with cross-sex hormones. *European Journal of Endocrinology, 164*(4), 635–642.

Blosnich, J. R., Brown, G. R., Shipherd J. C., Kauth, M., Piegari, R. I., & Bossarte, R. M. (2013). Prevalence of gender identity disorder and suicide risk among transgender veterans utilizing Veterans Health Administration care. *American Journal of Public Health, 103*(10), e27–32.

Blosnich, J. R., Brown, G. R., Wojcio, S., Jones, K. T., & Bossarte, R. M. (2014). Mortality among veterans with transgender-related diagnoses in the Veterans Health Administration, FY2000–2009. *LGBT Health, 1*(4), 269–276.

Bockting, W., Coleman, E., Deutsch, M. B., Guillamon, A., Meyer, I., Meyer, W., 3rd, . . . Ettner, R. (2016). Adult development and quality of life of transgender and gender nonconforming people. *Current Opinion in Endocrinology, Diabetes & Obesity, 23*(2), 188–197.

Brown, G. R., & Jones, K. T. (2015). Incidence of breast cancer in a cohort of 5,135 transgender veterans. *Breast Cancer Research and Treatment, 149*(1), 191–198.

Brown, G. R., & Jones, K. T. (2016). Mental health and medical health disparities in 5135 transgender veterans receiving healthcare in the Veterans Health Administration: A case-control study. *LGBT Health*, *3*(2), 122–131.

Byne, W. (2006). Developmental endocrine influences on gender identity: Implications for management of disorders of sex development. *Mount Sinai Journal of Medicine*, *73*(7), 950–959.

De Roo, C., Tilleman, K., T'Sjoen, G., & De Sutter, P. (2016). Fertility options in transgender people. *International Review of Psychiatry*, *28*(1), 112–119.

Dittrich, R., Binder, H., Cupisti, S., Hoffmann, I., Beckmann, M. W., & Mueller, A. (2005). Endocrine treatment of male-to-female transsexuals using gonadotropin-releasing hormone agonist. *Experimental and Clinical Endocrinology & Diabetes*, *113*(10), 586–592.

Esteva de Antonio, I., Gomez-Gil, E., & GIDSEEN Group (2013). Coordination of healthcare for transsexual persons: a multidisciplinary approach. *Current Opinion in Endocrinology, Diabetes & Obesity*, *20*(6), 585–591.

Fernandez-Balsells, M. M., Murad, M. H., Lane, M., Lampropulos, J. F., Albuquerque, F., Mullan, R. J., . . . Montori, V. M. (2010). Clinical review 1: Adverse effects of testosterone therapy in adult men: A systematic review and meta-analysis. *Journal of Clinical Endocrinology & Metabolism*, *95*(6), 2560–2575.

Gardner, I. H., & Safer, J. D. (2013). Progress on the road to better medical care for transgender patients. *Current Opinion in Endocrinology, Diabetes & Obesity*, *20*(6), 553–558.

Gooren, L. J. (2014). Management of female-to-male transgender persons: medical and surgical management, life expectancy. *Current Opinion in Endocrinology, Diabetes & Obesity*, *21*(3), 233–238.

Gooren, L. J., Giltay, E. J., & Bunck, M. C. (2008). Long-term treatment of transsexuals with cross-sex hormones: Extensive personal experience. *Journal of Clinical Endocrinology &Metabolism*, *93*(1), 19–25.

Gooren, L. J., van Trotsenburg, M. A., Giltay, E. J., & van Diest, P. J. (2013). Breast cancer development in transsexual subjects receiving cross-sex hormone treatment. *Journal of Sexual Medicine*, *10*(12), 3129–3134.

Gooren, L. J., Wierckx, K., & Giltay, E. J. (2014). Cardiovascular disease in transsexual persons treated with cross-sex hormones: Reversal of the traditional sex difference in cardiovascular disease pattern. *European Journal of Endocrinology*, *170*(6), 809–819.

Gurney, E. P., Nachtigall, M. J., Nachtigall, L. E., & Naftolin, F. (2014). The Women's Health Initiative trial and related studies: 10 years later: A clinician's view. *The Journal of Steroid Biochemistry and Molecular Biology*, *142*, 4–11.

Hembree, W. C., Cohen-Kettenis, P., Delemarre-van de Waal, H. A., Gooren, L. J., Meyer, W. J., 3rd, Spack, N. P., . . . Montori, V. M. (2009). Endocrine treatment of transsexual persons: An Endocrine Society clinical practice guideline. *Journal of Clinical Endocrinology & Metabolism*, *94*(9), 3132–3154.

Herbst, J. H., Jacobs, E. D., Finlayson, T. J., McKleroy, V. S., Neumann, M. S., & Crepaz, N. (2008). Estimating HIV prevalence and risk behaviors of transgender persons in the United States: a systematic review. *AIDS and Behavior*, *12*(1), 1–17.

Heylens, G., Elaut, E., Kreukels, B. P., Paap, M. C., Cerwenka, S., Richter-Appelt, H., . . . De Cuypere, G. (2014). Psychiatric characteristics in transsexual individuals: Multicentre study in four European countries. *The British Journal of Psychiatry*, *204*(2), 151–156.

Houk, C. P., & Lee, P. A. (2012). Update on disorders of sex development. *Current Opinion in Endocrinology, Diabetes & Obesity, 19*(1), 28–32.

Irwig, M. S. (2017). Testosterone therapy for transgender men. *The Lancet Diabetes & Endocrinology, 5*(4), 301–311.

Jacobeit, J. W., Gooren, L. J., & Schulte, H. M. (2009). Safety aspects of 36 months of administration of long-acting intramuscular testosterone undecanoate for treatment of female-to-male transgender individuals. *European Journal of Endocrinology, 161*(5), 795–798.

Johnson, L., Shipherd, J., & Walton, H. M. (2016). The psychologist's role in transgender-specific care with U.S. veterans. *Psychological Services, 13*(1), 69–76.

Kauth, M. R., Shipherd, J. C., Lindsay, J. A., Kirsh, S., Knapp, H., & Matza, L. (2015). Teleconsultation and training of VHA providers on transgender care: Implementation of a multisite hub system. *Telemedicine and e-Health, 21*(12), 1012–1018.

Klaver, M., Dekker, M. J., de Mutsert, R., Twisk, J. W., & den Heijer, M. (2016). Cross-sex hormone therapy in transgender persons affects total body weight, body fat and lean body mass: a meta-analysis. *Andrologia*. doi:10.1111/and.12660

Koulouri, O., & Conway, G. S. (2008). A systematic review of commonly used medical treatments for hirsutism in women. *Clinical Endocrinology (Oxford), 68*(5), 800–805.

Lapauw, B., Taes, Y., Simoens, S., Van Caenegem, E., Weyers, S., Goemaere, S., . . . T'Sjoen, G. G. (2008). Body composition, volumetric and areal bone parameters in male-to-female transsexual persons. *Bone, 43*(6), 1016–1021.

McCann, E., & Sharek, D. (2016). Mental health needs of people who identify as transgender: A review of the literature. *Archives of Psychiatric Nursing, 30*(2), 280–285.

McNeill, E. J. (2006). Management of the transgender voice. *The Journal of Laryngology & Otology, 120*(7), 521–523.

Mueck, A. O. (2012). Postmenopausal hormone replacement therapy and cardiovascular disease: The value of transdermal estradiol and micronized progesterone. *Climacteric, 15*(Supplement 1), 11–17. doi:10.3109/13697137.2012.669624

Neumann, M. S., Finlayson, T. J., Pitts, N. L., & Keatley, J. (2017). Comprehensive HIV prevention for transgender persons. *American Journal of Public Health, 107*(2), 207–212.

Nuttbrock, L., Hwahng, S., Bockting, W., Rosenblum, A., Mason, M., Macri, M., & Becker, J. (2009). Lifetime risk factors for HIV/sexually transmitted infections among male-to-female transgender persons. *Journal of Acquired Immune Deficiency Syndrome, 52*(3), 417–421.

Olié, V., Canonico, M., & Scarabin, P. Y. (2010). Risk of venous thrombosis with oral versus transdermal estrogen therapy among postmenopausal women. *Current Opinion in Hematology, 17*(5), 457–463.

Operario, D., Soma, T., & Underhill, K. (2008). Sex work and HIV status among transgender women: Systematic review and meta-analysis. *Journal of Acquired Immune Deficiency Syndrome, 48*(1), 97–103.

Oskui, P. M., French, W. J., Herring, M. J., Mayeda, G. S., Burstein, S., & Kloner, R. A. (2013). Testosterone and the cardiovascular system: a comprehensive review of the clinical literature. *Journal of the American Heart Association, 2*(6), e000272. doi:10.1161/jaha.113.000272

Pope, H. G., Jr., Kouri, E. M., & Hudson, J. I. (2000). Effects of supraphysiologic doses of testosterone on mood and aggression in normal men: A randomized controlled trial. *Archives of General Psychiatry, 57*(2), 133–140; discussion 155–156.

Prior, J. C., Vigna, Y. M., & Watson, D. (1989). Spironolactone with physiological female steroids for presurgical therapy of male-to-female transsexualism. *Archives of Sexual Behavior, 18*(1), 49–57.
Reisner, S. L., Poteat, T., Keatley, J., Cabral, M., Mothopeng, T., Dunham, E., . . . Baral, S. D. (2016). Global health burden and needs of transgender populations: A review. *The Lancet, 388*(10042), 412–436.
Rose, L. I., Underwood, R. H., Newmark, S. R., Kisch, E. S., & Williams, G. H. (1977). Pathophysiology of spironolactone-induced gynecomastia. *Annals of Internal Medicine, 87*(4), 398–403.
Shipherd, J. C., Kauth, M. R., & Matza, A. (2016). Nationwide interdisciplinary e-consultation on transgender care in the Veterans Health Administration. *Telemedicine and e-Health, 22*(12), 1008–1012.
Siu, A. L. (2015). Behavioral and pharmacotherapy interventions for tobacco smoking cessation in adults, including pregnant women: U.S. Preventive Services Task Force Recommendation Statement. *Annals of Internal Medicine, 163*(8), 622–634.
Weinand, J. D., & Safer, J. D. (2015). Hormone therapy in transgender adults is safe with provider supervision: A review of hormone therapy sequelae for transgender individuals. *Journal of Clinical and Translational Endocrinology, 2*(2), 55–60.
Wierckx, K., Elaut, E., Declercq, E., Heylens, G., De Cuypere, G., Taes, Y., . . . T'Sjoen, G. (2013). Prevalence of cardiovascular disease and cancer during cross-sex hormone therapy in a large cohort of trans persons: A case-control study. *European Journal of Endocrinology, 169*(4), 471–478.
Wilczynski, C., & Emanuele, M. A. (2014). Treating a transgender patient: Overview of the guidelines. *Postgraduate Medicine, 126*(7), 121–128. doi:10.3810/pgm.2014.11.2840
Winter, S., Diamond, M., Green, J., Karasic, D., Reed, T., Whittle, S., & Wylie, K. (2016). Transgender people: Health at the margins of society. *The Lancet, 388*(10042), 390–400.
World Professional Association for Transgender Health. (2011). *Standards of care for transsexual, transgender, and gender nonconforming people, Version* 7 (7th ed.). Retrieved from https://s3.amazonaws.com/amo_hub_content/Association140/files/Standards%20of%20Care%20V7%20-%202011%20WPATH%20(2)(1).pdf
Wylie, K., Knudson, G., Khan, S. I., Bonierbale, M., Watanyusakul, S., & Baral, S. (2016). Serving transgender people: clinical care considerations and service delivery models in transgender health. *The Lancet, 388*(10042), 401–411.

7 The High-Risk Client

Comorbid Conditions That Affect Care

Colleen A. Sloan, PhD
Joshua D. Safer, MS, FACP

The views expressed in this material are those of the authors and do not reflect the official policy or position of the Department of Veterans Affairs or the U.S. Government.

As described in Chapter 3, transgender people experience higher rates of mental health problems including depression, substance use, and suicidality, as well as increased rates of exposure to trauma compared to cisgender people (whose gender identity is congruent with their sex assigned at birth). Transgender clients may also present with significant difficulties regulating emotions and behavior (see Chapter 8), which may manifest via high-risk behavior, challenging interpersonal styles (e.g., demanding behavior) and extreme emotional lability, all of which can potentially pose problems in gaining access to care, establishing therapeutic rapport, making progress in treatment, and achieving goals including those specific to gender transitioning (Richmond, Burnes, & Carroll, 2012). As such, these problems have the capacity to further promote disparities for an already marginalized population, particularly within health care settings. Moreover, increased experience with stigma, prejudice, and discrimination could potentially exacerbate the aforementioned mental health problems and presentations, thus making treatment less feasible and effective. For example, a client who experiences discrimination and hostility in their daily lives will likely approach the health care setting with suspicion and an expectation of harm. It is the responsibility of the mental health professional to create a safe and welcoming environment that normalizes this experience and facilitates progress despite that stance. Often it can be helpful to simply acknowledge that trust is earned and that the provider is motivated to earn the trust of the client.

High-Risk Mental and Behavioral Health Problems Affecting Transgender Clients

Within the United States (U.S.), the Diagnostic and Statistical Manual for Mental Health Disorders, Fifth Edition (DSM-5; American Psychiatric Association [APA], 2013), uses Gender Dysphoria as the mental health diagnosis that captures distress regarding the incongruence between one's sex assigned at birth and one's gender identity, whereas the 10th revision of the International Statistical Classification of Diseases and Related Health Problems (ICD), a medical classification list by the World Health Organization (WHO), uses the mental health diagnosis Gender Identity Disorder (World Health Organization, 1993). The DSM-5 identifies anxiety and depressive disorders as commonly co-occurring with Gender Dysphoria, and suggests that, as a consequence of increased nonacceptance of gender non-conforming behavior over time, these co-occurring disorders seem to increase with age (APA, 2013). The available literature has revealed alarming statistics, most notably significantly elevated rates of suicidality in transgender individuals (for a review see Haas et al., 2011). Results from the most recent United States Transgender Survey (U.S.T.S.), which included 27,715 respondents from all 50 states, revealed that roughly 40% of transgender respondents had attempted suicide in their lifetime, a rate nearly nine times the rate of the U.S. population (James et al., 2016).

In a study examining suicidal behavior in transgender youth, investigators found that over half of the sample reported having engaged in a life-threatening behavior, while roughly one fourth reported actually having attempted suicide (Grossman & D'Augelli, 2007). Similar rates have been found in a young adult sample, and these results also highlighted the unique association between gender-based discrimination and gender-based victimization on suicide attempts (Clements-Nolle, Marx, & Katz, 2006). Strikingly high rates have been found in transgender veteran samples, with results showing rates 20 times higher for transgender veterans when compared to cisgender veterans (Blosnich et al., 2013), and they die at a younger age compared with their veteran peers (Blosnich, Brown, Wojcio, Jones, & Bossarte, 2014).

Suicidality notwithstanding, other concerning issues have been noted in transgender communities, including high-risk sexual behavior, homelessness, and engagement in sex work (Herbst et al., 2008; Wilson et al., 2009), as well as substance use problems (Hughes & Eliason, 2002). It has been suggested that substance use functions as a means to cope with transgender-related stigma and discrimination, at least in a subset of the transgender population (Bockting, 2014; Hendricks & Testa, 2012; Reisner et al., 2015). Additionally, recent data taken from a large online study of transgender individuals indicated a high prevalence of depression, anxiety, and somatization (Bockting et al., 2013).

Another recent study investigating mental health problems in transgender veterans found increased rates of depression, serious mental illness, and posttraumatic stress disorder (PTSD; Brown & Jones, 2015a). Results from the U.S.T.S. further support these findings, indicating higher rates of discrimination, HIV, homelessness, poverty, unemployment, especially for transgender women of color, when compared to the U.S. population (James et al., 2016). Collectively, these findings demonstrate health disparities for transgender clients, as well as a relationship between experiences of discrimination and poor mental health in transgender people over and above experiences of Gender Dysphoria. Chapter 8 presents a conceptualization and treatment approach for gender-related distress and associated mental health problems in transgender clients. The remainder of the current chapter will provide recommendations for targeting specific risk factors that may interfere with effective treatment for gender dysphoria, particularly hormone therapy.

Recommendations for Treatment When Working with High-Risk Transgender Clients

As mentioned in previous chapters, effective treatment for transgender clients, particularly those pursuing a gender transition, generally comprises an interdisciplinary approach. Therefore, mental health professionals working with transgender clients are likely to be most effective and feel most supported if working within an interdisciplinary team. However, this is often not the case, making working alone much more challenging. Regardless of theoretical orientation, training, and education, mental health professionals are likely to be more effective when working with high-risk transgender clients via utilization of a skills-based approach to treatment, balancing both acceptance- and change-based strategies. A skills-based approach functions to assist transgender clients to more effectively cope with stressors, whether those stressors are directly related to their transgender identity or not, and navigate their worlds competently. Moreover, a skills-based approach to treatment can be easily learned and utilized by all mental health professionals regardless of their background and training, which assists in increasing access to care for transgender clients.

Interventions for the treatment of Gender Dysphoria (in DSM-5; APA, 2013) or Gender Identity Disorder (in ICD-10; WHO, 1993), which may or may not be present for a transgender person, are generally change-based (e.g., alteration of gender expression, hormone therapy, and surgical interventions). However, these interventions may not be effective in reducing high-risk behavior. Moreover, these interventions may not function to achieve desired outcomes or may not be available (e.g., due to financial strain or medical contraindications). Therefore, solely focusing or relying on medical interventions is inadequate. As mentioned previously, quality transgender care is interdisciplinary, and understanding a client's medical risk profile is important for mental health professionals to be able to effectively assist a client in weighing the cost/benefit ratios of various treatments. Equally important is the mental health provider's role as teacher and coach for new skill development, so a transgender client can interact more effectively with medical providers, and at work and in social settings. These roles can also be balanced by connecting clients to peer support groups and other validating spaces (see Chapters 8 and 10).

Change-based behavioral skills are recommended to assist and support transgender clients in coping with a variety of stressors. Examples of change-based skills include assertiveness training (e.g., Paterson, 2000; Smith, 1975), pleasant events scheduling/engagement, problem-solving, self-care, and cognitive skills. Examples of contexts in which assertiveness training would be particularly beneficial include advocating for health care services, making requests from others regarding preferred name and pronouns, and managing legal issues including requests for changes to identity documents. Pleasant events scheduling and engagement are designed to assist with improving mood, which in turn can promote risk reduction and can specifically encourage solicitation of social support, particularly within the transgender community. Self-care can be particularly challenging for high-risk clients, especially for those who are homeless or have inadequate housing and those with restricted finances irrespective of housing status. As such, collaboratively working to identify ways to improve self-care is important to assist with overall health and reduce vulnerability to mental and physical health problems. Lastly, cognitive skills, including cognitive modification, is likely to foster objective evaluation of physical (e.g., "safe" spaces for transgender people) and medical risk (e.g., "doubling my dose of hormones will double the effects"), generation of balanced ways of thinking about gender transition (e.g., realistic outcomes based on facts), as well as with challenging potentially rigid and/or dichotomous beliefs about gender and gender roles (e.g., "I'm not a real woman unless I have breasts."). As with any skills-based teaching/learning, skills improve with practice. Therefore, treatment effectiveness may be enhanced via modeling, participation in role-plays, coaching, and/or otherwise directly supported use of skills.

Suicidality

As noted earlier, rates of suicidal behavior are strikingly high for the transgender population. While an abundance of literature exists on the topic of suicide in the general population, less has focused on suicide in the transgender population. Moreover, research exclusively focusing on effective interventions for suicide has been sparse. Linehan and colleagues (2012) highlighted that the number of clinical trials that focus on targeting suicidal behavior in the general population is also strikingly low. The number of clinical trials focusing on reduction of suicidal behavior in the transgender population is zero, despite ample evidence of increased suicide rates in this population (e.g., Blosnich et al., 2013). The Linehan (2012) article contains an appendix to assist clinicians in the assessment and management of suicide risk, which includes review of risk and protective factors, as well as specific safety planning components. Thus, it offers a place to start when working with suicidal transgender clients.

Cognitive-Behavioral Therapy for Suicidal Behavior

Effective risk assessment and management is paramount in the treatment of suicidal behavior. Thorough assessment allows providers to determine the most appropriate type and level of care for suicidal individuals. The recommended comprehensive approach to effective treatment of suicidality comprises multiple components, including some or all of the following: hospitalization (for acute threats to life), psychopharmacotherapy, intensive case management, risk management, and outpatient mental health care specifically aimed at reducing/addressing risk factors and improving overall quality of life. For transgender clients, the idea of engaging with inpatient and/or residential treatment can be particularly challenging as clients will need clear information about where they will be housed (ideally based on gender identity, not birth sex) and what protections will be offered to them should they encounter harassment or discrimination by staff or other residents. To facilitate this type of admission, effective coordination of care is necessary, which will require an initial investment of time by the mental health provider in order to both review the inpatient setting processes and level of knowledge (ideally happening in advance of acute need) and to fully inform the transgender client and minimize the risks for the admission. Mental health professionals are encouraged to work closely with local inpatient programs and assure that staff members have received appropriate training on transgender health and safety issues for their milieu.

Safety planning is of utmost importance when care is restricted or limited when working with suicidal transgender individuals. Stanley and Brown (2012) describe a brief, stand-alone intervention for the reduction of suicide risk and associated behavior, which can be applied to transgender clients. They outline key components of effective safety planning, which includes: recognition of warning signs (gleaned during risk assessment); employment of internal coping strategies; utilization of social support for: 1) distraction from suicidal thoughts, 2) assistance in management of crises, and 3) seeking out of mental health professional support; and means restriction (Stanley & Brown, 2012).

More specifically related to internal coping strategies, a cognitive-behavioral approach to treatment aims specifically to identify maladaptive beliefs that encourage and maintain problematic emotional (e.g., depression) and behavioral patterns (e.g., suicide) and to identify ways in which problematic behavior (e.g., sleeping during the day) reinforces maladaptive beliefs (e.g., "I'm worthless"). A cognitive-behavioral therapy (CBT) approach specifically aims to change maladaptive beliefs (e.g., cognitive therapy for depression; Beck, Rush, Shaw, & Emery, 1979; Beck, 1995) and problematic behavioral patterns (e.g., behavioral activation for depression; Jacobson et al., 1996; Jacobson, Martell, & Dimidjian, 2001).

Wenzel and colleagues (2009) authored a comprehensive book titled, *Cognitive Therapy for Suicidal Patients: Scientific and Clinical Applications*, in which they present an extensive review of factors related to suicidal behavior. These factors apply to suicidal transgender clients. The authors offer a cognitive case conceptualization model of suicidal behavior, methods of assessment, and describe cognitive interventions. Specifically, the authors discuss "core beliefs" or "schemas" that are likely to develop and surface in suicidal individuals—trait hopelessness and unbearability (Wenzel & Beck, 2008; Wenzel et al., 2009). Wenzel suggests that when these "schemas" are activated, they can contribute to a sense of overwhelming hopelessness, which in turn encourages attentional bias/constriction, thus reducing objective evaluation of incoming information. Moreover, this attentional constriction significantly interferes with problem-solving capabilities, which increases the likelihood that suicide will be considered as an option (Wenzel et al., 2009). Therefore, treatment will include first identification of problematic thinking patterns, questions that inherently challenge these thoughts, evaluation of evidence for and against these thoughts, and generation of alternative thoughts that function to reduce the sense of hopelessness and increase tolerance (i.e., bearability).

For example, suppose a young transgender girl (i.e., male sex assigned at birth and female gender identity) begins secretly dressing in traditionally female clothing, perhaps borrowing from her sister or mother. Her father learns of this behavior, and severely punishes her, communicating a strong message that this gender "non-conforming" behavior is not acceptable. This experience may lead to an increased sense of hopelessness, given that the young girl now has encoded messages that something is inherently "wrong" with her, and she has no access to strategies that assist with reducing gender dysphoric feelings. Now suppose that a few years later, this young girl undergoes puberty and begins developing male secondary sex characteristics, leading to increased dysphoria and an increased sense of unbearability of her physical body and associated masculine gender role that is encouraged by her parents, particularly her father. The more unbearable her situation feels to her, the more likely she is to decide that she can no longer live as a boy. She discloses to her parents that she is a girl and would like to undergo a gender transition. Her parents force her out of their home, and she begins living on the street at age 14. Without any resources, she becomes increasingly hopeless. While living on the streets, she is assaulted, arrested, and incarcerated in a male juvenile detention center, further increasing her sense of hopelessness and unbearability. With seemingly no viable options or access to positive support or coping, she believes her only option is suicide.

Homelessness, Sex Work, and Other High-Risk Sexual Behavior

As previously mentioned, care for high-risk transgender clients ideally utilizes an interdisciplinary approach. This is especially effective when clients present with many needs most suitable for case management services, as is likely the case for transgender clients who are homeless and/or unemployed. As such, mental health professionals may either provide case management services directly or refer clients for these services, working collaboratively with other health care providers. If the former, it is imperative to become familiar with and knowledgeable about local resources and their sensitivity to transgender clients' needs. For example, it is likely beneficial to reach out directly to local programs, organizations, and facilities, particularly those that offer resources for homelessness. If work with transgender clients is new, mental health providers may make these contacts on clients' behalf, at least initially to determine policies, practices, and procedures around transgender issues. This work is important as a breach in trust would occur if referring your client to programs or shelters that do not have adequate protections.

Concomitantly, a long-term goal is to also work with clients to develop skills to advocate on their own behalf, which may or may not necessitate additional advocacy directly from providers. When initiating contact with homeless shelters, residential programs, or any other service, it will be important to first assess factors that will likely prove challenging for transgender people. These factors include but are not limited to bathroom facilities, patient protection policies that explicitly mention gender identity and/or gender expression, general organization of facilities (e.g., gendered spaces; private spaces), and sleeping arrangements (e.g., occupants segregated by gender, not birth sex), as well as weapons and substance use policies and security. For example, some homeless shelters are "wet" shelters, which allow occupants to reside with possession of substances and/or reside while under the influence of substances. Transgender clients who are struggling to manage sobriety may be more effectively housed in "dry" shelters, which do not allow substances on the premises and do not allow occupants to reside while under the influence. However, if a "wet" shelter has more transgender affirming policies (e.g., access to bathrooms consistent with gender identity), then mental health professionals can work with their transgender clients to develop effective coping plans to manage substance use urges, etc.

Ideally, resources including case management, housing, and substance use treatment programs that are readily available and have transgender affirming policies. However, as mentioned previously, this is often not the case. Consequently, mental health professionals may need to "step outside of comfort zones" and provide services that are traditionally provided by other disciplines (e.g., case management) and/or develop consultation skills to work with local agencies to create more welcoming environments at existing local agencies where needed programs are located. Mental health professionals may find themselves targeting a host of problems in the absence of additional support. Mental health providers are encouraged to utilize a harm-reduction (Luoma, Kohlenberg, Hayes, Bunting, & Rye, 2008; Marlatt, 1996; Marlatt & Tapert, 1993) approach to therapy, working with high-risk transgender clients to target risk hierarchically: for example, prioritizing risk-factors like homelessness (Tsemberis, Gulcur, & Nakae, 2004) and high-risk behavior (e.g., drug use; Springer, 1992) that can contribute to further health disparities (e.g., HIV/AIDS).

Managing Extreme Behavior/Demanding Clients

When clients present with extreme and/or demanding behavior, this has many potential consequences for mental health and medical treatment. First, this behavior can negatively affect therapeutic alliance, which can disrupt and/or delay access to treatment. Clinicians may feel little to no motivation to assist transgender clients who present with challenging interpersonal styles. Second, demanding behavior may also be secondary to a strong sense of urgency to access care, utilize therapies, and make progress in gender transition. This sense of urgency coupled with a perception of health care providers as "gatekeepers to care" can naturally result in clients presenting as angry and upset. While a sense of urgency may make sense given distress and desire for change, collaborating with clients to define and achieve goals while also gently challenging clients' demanding behavior may be necessary to assist with realistic goal-setting and getting (valid) needs met. As mentioned above, a skills-based approach to therapy is likely beneficial, in addition to validation strategies as discussed in Chapter 8.

Mental Health Considerations When Working with Transgender Elders

Transgender elders have been identified as a particularly at-risk, underserved, and understudied group (e.g., Fredriksen-Goldsen et al., 2014; Persson, 2009), both within the transgender health and gerontology/geropsychology literatures. While transgender elders may share similarities with their cisgender elder counterparts regarding ageing and end-of-life concerns, they also have unique experiences and health care needs, which complicates an already challenging developmental stage (Williams & Freeman, 2007). As such, the available gerontological literature provides minimal information regarding the unique needs of this community, as well as limited guidance on effective interventions for mental and behavioral health problems that may exist for older transgender clients (Kimmel, 2014). Moreover, transgender elders are also unique from younger cohorts of transgender people, by virtue of their having lived through a broad and diverse transgender history, spanning a time that began with almost complete invisibility of transgender experiences to the present time in which transgender identities and experiences are quite visible (Cook-Daniels, 2016). This unique history contributes to wide variability regarding the individual experiences of transgender older adults. Mental health professionals should engage in open-ended questioning when inquiring about these unique experiences and should avoid making assumptions and/or generalizations regarding the individual journeys of their clients (Cook-Daniels, 2016).

Transgender elders, like their younger cohorts and LGB elders, also evidence increased rates of mental health problems and experiences of discrimination (e.g., Fredriksen-Goldsen et al., 2014; Porter et al., 2016; Witten, 2014), but also evidence poorer mental and physical health and higher rates of discrimination when compared to their cisgender sexual minority counterparts (Fredriksen-Goldsen et al., 2014). Moreover, given the wide variability of individual experiences across the life span, transgender elders may present at various points during their gender transitions or may have opted not to transition at all. Mental health professionals should learn about each individual client's unique reasons for their decision-making and should be prepared to help clients manage emotions around such decision-making. For example, transgender clients may experience feelings of resentment or regret for having not transitioned, may have a strong sense of urgency to capitalize on an opportunity to transition later in life or alternatively may opt to "detransition" out of fear of discrimination in long-term care facilities (Cook-Daniels, 2016; Porter et al., 2016; Witten, 2014). Mental health professionals can assist transgender clients to effectively solve complex problems and evaluate decisions by engaging in open discussion regarding costs and benefits and working to help transgender clients cope with apparent costs. With this in mind, treatment may focus on processing and managing grief and other losses that accompany difficult decisions. Relatedly, transgender elders may have reasonable fears that they will die having been disrespected (e.g., buried in a manner that reflects their sex assigned at birth; Witten, 2014). Mental health professionals can work with clients to engage in effective planning to ensure that end-of-life wishes are carried out.

Much of the available literature on transgender elder health encourages mental health professionals to focus on resilience with their clients (e.g., Porter et al., 2016; Witten, 2014). Indeed, several modifiable risk factors have been identified including stigma, victimization, health-related behaviors, and social support (Fredriksen-Goldsen et al., 2014). Therefore, mental health professionals should work collaboratively with their transgender elder clients to target these factors, which may include behavior modification regarding health behavior and support in utilizing health care, as transgender elders may avoid seeking health care due to past negative experiences (e.g., Cook-Daniels, 2016). Moreover, mental health professionals can advocate on behalf of and/or with their clients to target potential discrimination evident in institutional settings in which transgender elders may live, such as assisted living facilities. Lastly, and importantly, mental health professionals should actively work with transgender clients to seek out and connect with social support, as this has been identified as a pertinent protective factor as well as encouraging active engagement in values-based activities (Fredriksen-Goldsen et al., 2014; Porter et al., 2016).

Considerations for Hormone Therapy

Chapter 6 discussed ways to effectively prepare clients for hormone therapy. When transgender clients present with high-risk problems, careful attention must be paid to the hormone therapy regimens, as health risks are potentially increased. Relatedly, clients who have other mental health problems in addition to gender dysphoria and/or increased psychosocial stressors may have difficulty utilizing hormone therapy effectively. The next section will discuss high-risk conditions that affect hormone therapy as well as strategies for mitigating risk, keeping the non-prescribing mental health professional in mind.

Primary Hormone Therapy Risks and Strategies

Compiled evidence suggests that hormone therapy for transgender individuals is safe without a large risk of adverse events when followed carefully for a few well-documented medical concerns (Weinand & Safer, 2015). Unfortunately, it is all too common that transgender individuals use the Internet to self-prescribe "natural remedies" and black market hormones. The major risks of such sources are that the products will not contain the hormones desired or that they will contain other agents with unknown safety profiles. Even if the products supplied are genuine, self-treatment does not include appropriate monitoring and puts the individuals in danger of under-dosage, over-dosage, and insidious side effects.

The primary concern among transgender women on estrogen therapy is the possibility of developing thrombogenic complications (blood clots) like deep venous thrombosis (in limbs), pulmonary embolism (lungs), and stroke (Asscheman et al., 2014; Gooren, Giltay, & Bunck, 2008; Lehrman, 1976; Wierckx et al., 2012; Wierckx et al., 2013). Therefore, educating transgender women and their providers regarding preventative ways to minimize risk of thromboembolic events might be the most important long-term intervention (many of them behavioral) to minimize the risk of adverse effects from estrogen. Coordination of care between mental health professionals and medical providers is key.

Suggested risk modifications from groups studying venous thrombo-embolism (VTE) among transgender women include addressing high cholesterol, high blood pressure, and smoking. Much of this work can be done with mental health professionals who offer a behavioral medicine approach to reducing risks through behavioral interventions such as diet, exercise, and smoking cessation programs. Interventions to help with smoking cessation, including medical interventions (e.g., Chantix®), are not known to interact with reproductive hormones. They are anticipated to be as safe in transgender individuals as in the general population. Although some advocate complete discontinuation of estrogen in transgender women with histories of thrombotic events, greater experience has some medical practitioners following the protocols for women in general with anti-coagulation regimens as needed in order to maintain the hormone treatment regimen. However, this type of calculated risk can only occur with a client who is compliant with medication and lab monitoring. Thus, the role of the mental health professional in assisting the client in understanding the cost/benefit ratio of this approach and level of commitment to medication schedules and monitoring is invaluable. Other health concerns that require monitoring for transgender women taking hormones may include increased triglycerides (Meyer et al., 1986) and decreased sexual desire (Wierckx et al., 2014). See Chapter 13 for additional detail about sexual health.

Even complicated medical comorbidities are not always considered absolute contraindications to hormone therapy (e.g., predisposition to thromboembolism). However, it may still be the case that some clients and their medical providers will collaboratively decide that risk from a preferred hormone treatment strategy is greater than is acceptable. For example, a client may discontinue estrogen due to thrombosis risk or determine that a surgery including gonadectomy is preferred to the current hormone regimen.

The primary concern among transgender men on testosterone therapy results from the well-established erythropoiesis stimulation by androgens (Weinand & Safer, 2015). That is, testosterone and other androgens stimulate the growth of red blood cells (erythropoiesis). The two classic tests that may assess this are hematocrit and/or hemoglobin. Increased hematocrit (the percentage of a person's blood that is solid red blood cells rather than liquid) means increased oxygen carrying capacity. However, if the hematocrit is too high, it becomes a clotting risk. Therefore, the primary monitoring for transgender men on testosterone therapy is hematocrit to ascertain that dosing does not result in a dangerous rise to greater than 55% per Endocrine Society Guidelines (Hembree et al., 2009), but in the absence of data some authors use 50% as a limit with some cushion (Gardner & Safer, 2013). Dose adjustments and other interventions (e.g., phlebotomy) are sometimes required to achieve safe hematocrit levels.

It is rare to have an absolute contraindication to testosterone therapy. The harms from the absence of testosterone usually outweigh the concerns regarding exacerbation of medical morbidities. The classic contraindication to testosterone therapy for cisgender men is prostate malignancy, which does not apply to transgender men. For transgender women, alternatives to hormone therapy may be indicated including surgical procedures, such as orchiectomy, which reduces necessity of feminizing hormone therapy. For other transgender clients, it may still be the case that they and their medical providers will make the decision that risk from a preferred hormone treatment strategy is greater than is acceptable. For example, a client may discontinue testosterone due to uncontrolled polycythemia (elevated hematocrit). In situations such as these, mental health professionals can actively work with clients to cope with emotions that may arise in the context of this loss. Painful emotions are likely to arise when important objectives and goals of a gender transition are blocked, delayed, or otherwise not available. Mental health professionals can help transgender clients validate their own emotional responses, while simultaneously working to increase acceptance and tolerance of painful realities. Chapter 8 discusses possible applications of acceptance-based strategies when working with transgender clients.

Other Hormone Therapy Risk Considerations

Both feminizing and masculinizing treatments have been reported to worsen control of blood sugars over time and increase risk of developing diabetes (Jacobeit, Gooren, & Schulte, 2009; Resmini et al., 2008; Wierckx et al., 2012; Wierckx et al., 2013; Yamauchi et al., 2001). Whether the risk is due to hormone treatment or simply a part of ageing is not known. However, it would be prudent for transgender clients to anticipate when initiating hormone treatment. Mental health professionals can assist transgender clients to develop and engage in behavior modification programs to reduce this risk.

Although modest, current research supports the view that there is no significant increase in cancer prevalence among transgender individuals on hormone therapy (Brown & Jones, 2015b; Jacobeit, Gooren, & Schulte, 2009; Kuroda, Ohnisi, Sakamoto, & Itoyama, 2008; Miller, Bedard, Cooter, & Shaul, 1986; Wierckx et al., 2012). Specifically, although older guidelines suggested a cancer risk for transgender men with intact female reproductive tract tissues, the majority of current research does not show a reason to anticipate such a risk (Baldassarre et al., 2013; Dorff, Shazer, Nepomuceno, & Tucker, 2007; Gardner, Safer, Mok, Weiss, & Kuohong, 2014; Ikeda et al., 2012; Mikhaĭlichenko et al., 2013; Turo, Jallad, Prescott, & Cross, 2013). The result is that decisions for hysterectomy for transgender men have become very personal decisions to be worked out between the client and physician, and mental health professionals should be prepared to support clients with those conversations and decisions. Independent of specific risk, all transgender individuals must have plans in place to monitor all tissues present for cancer risk over time, regardless of the sex with which those tissues are typically associated.

Transgender individuals should also not exclude surveillance for cancers related to any tissues present; transgender women who have had genital reconstruction surgery (vaginoplasty) have presented with prostate cancer, and transgender men with uterine and cervical cancer (Bergoglio et al., 2013; Gooren & Morgenthaler, 2014; Pattison & McLaren, 2013; Pritchard, Pankowsky, Crowe, & Abdul-Karim, 1988). Both transgender women and transgender men have presented with breast cancer (Bowman et al., 2012; Deipolyi, Han, & Parsa, 2010; Dhand & Dhaliwal, 2010; Ganly & Taylor, 1995; Grabellus et al., 2005; Shao, Grossbard, & Klein, 2011; Symmers, 1968; Urban, Teng, & Kapp, 2011).

Except for a few large cohort and long-term studies, much of the existing knowledge about the health impact of transgender hormone therapy is based on case reports. While these provide clues to the effects of transgender hormone treatments, there is a strong need for future research of greater cohort size to be undertaken in order to address this critical gap.

Surgical Interventions

For a thorough discussion of transition-related surgical interventions, see Chapter 9. Transgender surgical interventions can be divided into three broad categories: 1) facial surgeries (usually facial feminization surgeries for transgender women); 2) chest reconstruction surgeries (removal of tissue and reconstruction for transgender men; breast augmentation for transgender women); and 3) genital tract surgeries (e.g., vaginoplasty, orchiectomy for transgender women; hysterectomy, oophorectomy, metoidioplasty, phalloplasty for transgender men). Transgender individuals undergoing surgery of any sort will need a stable safe environment in which to recover with recovery times varying from weeks to months. After the acute period of recovery, clients will need to be in a position to follow precise wound care instructions and to have physical help if that is necessary. Mental health professionals should proactively work with transgender clients to target post-surgical planning, particularly when working with clients who are homeless or elderly.

It is imperative for mental health professionals and medical providers to be keenly aware of any potential risk of transgender women clients engaging (or having urges/plans to engage) in auto-castration, as this significantly increases risk of harm and accidental death. Mental health professionals should aim for prevention and engage in open discussion regarding these types of urges, validating distress associated with gender dysphoric feelings around genitalia, and coaching clients on effectively managing urges via skills use. Chapter 8 discusses possible applications of change- and acceptance-based skills to help transgender clients cope with problematic behavioral urges, as well as cope and recover within challenging environments (e.g., shelters, assisted living facilities).

In addition to general postsurgical considerations, transgender individuals undergoing more involved genital tract surgeries (specifically, vaginoplasty and phalloplasty) must be in a reasonable position to follow detailed post-operative care instructions for their lifetimes. Transgender women who have had vaginoplasty will need to use a dilator system daily (and more frequently in the immediate postoperative period) if the goal is to maintain a patent vagina. Transgender men who have had a phalloplasty must be in a position to provide self-care if there are complications like strictures of the urethra (scarring that can cause blockage). Most plastic surgeons will insist on strict medical criteria for patients undergoing genital surgeries. Criteria may include age cut-offs, body mass index (BMI) limits (BMI is the standard measure of degree of obesity), diabetes limits (either that diabetes be controlled or that the patient not have diabetes), and complete cessation of tobacco use permanently. Medical interventions to assist patients with these may be considered.

As mentioned earlier, there are no transgender-hormone-associated contraindications to the use of any smoking cessation product, any conventional weight loss regimen, or any diabetes treatment agent. Mental health professionals should work collaboratively with transgender clients to identify ways to practice behavior that supports effective postoperative care and lifetime regimens. While this work may begin in the context of mental health treatment, professionals should work with clients to move toward independent engagement in such behavior to promote long-term functioning and individual competency.

Case Examples

1. Tamara is a 31-year-old bi-racial, Latina transgender woman. She has been "out" as transgender since the age of 16, at which time her family disowned her. Tamara has either been homeless or with inadequate housing since age 17. She is unemployed and has a long history of engaging in sex work dating back to late adolescence. This ultimately led to Tamara contracting HIV, which is not well managed at present. Recently, Tamara was assaulted while walking home from a bar and suffered severe physical injuries, which led to an emergency room admission. During the admission, Tamara voiced hopelessness and suicidal ideation to one of her providers, which prompted a psychiatric referral and mental health assessment.

   Tamara endorses many mental health symptoms, including those consistent with depression, anxiety, and PTSD and problematic substance use. She describes her life as "a mess" and states that it has "always been this way." She endorses a history of suicidal behavior, marked by at least two serious attempts, the first of which occurred at age 22. She has been psychiatrically hospitalized four times and reports that she has sought hospitalization when "feeling like [she] can't take life anymore." Regarding gender transitioning, Tamara has been using feminizing hormones, which she has been purchasing from transgender women friends for the past ten years. She states that she sometimes will "use a little extra when feeling down." She would like to pursue surgical interventions including facial feminization surgery and gender confirmation surgery. However, she has no insurance and does not know when these interventions will be possible for her. She has received silicone injections from a friend to assist with breast augmentation.

   Tamara reports a childhood history significant for verbal and emotional abuse from both parents and physical abuse from her father. She also endorses having been bullied throughout her childhood and adolescence including verbal and physical aggression. Her parents were largely unsupportive and stated that she could have avoided this victimization if she "just acted like a boy." As an adult, she has been sexually assaulted on multiple occasions.

   Tamara presents with many risk factors, most notably homelessness, sex work, HIV+ status, barriers to health care, and risky use of illicit hormones and non-medical breast augmentation. Collectively, all of these risk factors have contributed to increased hopelessness, resulting in suicidality. An ideal approach to treatment would entail care from multiple disciplines including case management, mental health, and primary care (and possibly endocrinology, although primary care may provide hormone therapy). Case management is likely to be particularly beneficial and should be prioritized to target homelessness and to connect Tamara with resources that may assist with access to health care (e.g., HIV treatment), safe employment, and other financial support. Adequate housing is likely to assist with overall stability, which may reduce hopelessness. Additionally, Tamara's risk of medical problems is increased due to her misuse of feminizing hormones and silicone injections. Only through a strong alliance with a team of health care providers will it be possible to suggest stopping with these interventions and connecting with appropriate treatment for Gender Dysphoria, HIV, and other comorbid conditions.

Relatedly, Tamara may also benefit from learning skills to cope with ongoing stressors. Importantly, Tamara may benefit from learning change-based strategies including cognitive modification skills to target schemas that give rise to suicidality (e.g., hopelessness and unbearability) and behavioral activation to target ongoing symptoms of depression. Behavioral activation exercises may include ways to increase social support and connection to the transgender community and communities of color. At the same time, it will be important to also emphasize acceptance-based strategies, especially given that Tamara is particularly marginalized in the intersectionality of her identities. As a result, Tamara may be challenged to identify supportive networks. Mental health providers may play a more active role, at least initially, in assisting Tamara to effectively utilize the above-mentioned resources, employ skills, and connect to social support. Over time, the goal is for Tamara to increase her use of skills independently, rely less on intensive resources, effectively manage physical health, and maintain reduction of gender dysphoria. Treatment of other comorbid conditions, including her PTSD and remaining anxiety and depression could also be of benefit.

2. Christine is a 65-year-old White transgender woman. She has been on transgender hormone treatment for 15 years following a conventional regimen that includes 4 mg of estradiol orally each day along with 200 mg of spironolactone each day. Her laboratory testing has been stable and at goal for years with her testosterone level in the female range and her potassium levels in a safe range on her current spironolactone dose. Because there were no local surgeons and insurance would not cover the procedure, Christine never had genital tract surgery and so has intact testes. Therefore, she is dependent on her medicine regimen to keep her levels in the female range.

   Christine's medical provider has told her that when the ovaries of a cisgender woman start to fail (menopause, at approximately age 50), it is usual practice to replace the lost estrogen with low doses only (typically 0.625 mg of conjugated estrogens or 0.5 mg of estradiol). Some women use estrogen patches in addition because that route of administration decreases clotting risk further. Were Christine to decrease her estrogen dose, however, her testosterone level would rise back toward or even into the male range with some masculinizing physical changes especially with regard to hair pattern. Christine discussed this information with her physician, and they agreed that because Christine's exposure to estrogen was far shorter than that of a cisgender woman, a case could be made for claiming a later menopause too. It was Christine's intention to have genital surgery including gonadectomy when it became available and then follow a typical post-menopause estrogen regimen.

Unfortunately, Christine is not very active, and she followed her family pattern for overweight, inactive members with development of diabetes mellitus as she aged. She has been unable to achieve optimal control and has a glycosylated hemoglobin of 8.5, with good control considered to be less than 7 (and normal less than 6, depending on the reference). Christine grew very excited a year ago when insurance started covering transgender medical care including surgery and a local surgical team started performing the vaginoplasty surgery that she wanted. Unfortunately, because of her age and diabetes, Christine cannot get on the waiting list for the surgery, and it is not clear that out-of-state surgeons would operate on her either with her current poor diabetes control.

Christine and her physician have discussed the current situation, which seems to mean an indefinite status quo without surgery for Christine. Christine has tentatively agreed with her physician that she should cut her estrogen dose to the usual post-menopausal dose even though it seems likely that she will then have a male level testosterone with associated changes developing. Christine's mental health provider should work with her collaboratively to objectively evaluate these options further. It may be possible that surgery would be available to Christine if her diabetes was well managed. With this in mind, Christine may work collaboratively with her mental health provider and her physician to develop a diet and exercise regimen with the explicit goal of effectively managing diabetes and increasing eligibility for surgery. However, if Christine chooses against this option (or if surgery is still not an option), and she moves forward with reduced estrogen dose, her mental health provider can assist her with coping with undesired male characteristics (e.g., hair pattern) and increasing acceptance that surgery is not available to her. Relatedly, Christine may also learn effective coping strategies that manage any distress related to presence of male secondary sex characteristics (e.g., genitalia). Should Christine's dysphoria increase with the reduced estrogen and she does not feel able to cope with undesired male characteristics, or if depression or suicidality emerge, an increase in her estrogen could be discussed with her physician.

Take Home Points

- Transgender and gender non-conforming clients are at increased risk for mental health and medical problems.
- Moving beyond these disparities will necessarily entail advocacy on the part of mental health (and other) professionals providing care to transgender clients, particularly those who are considered high-risk.
- Mental health professionals are encouraged to seek out training and education opportunities to learn more about transgender health in particular, as well as interventions (ideally evidence-based) for the comorbid conditions discussed within this chapter and other chapters of this book.
- Mental health professionals should also become educated regarding medical risk factors as well, even if they are not prescribers, and work with transgender clients to modify risk factors to the degree possible.
- Ageing transgender individuals may need to discontinue medical therapy at some point and mental health professionals can help these clients cope with that loss.
- Mental health professionals may need to help previously successfully treated transgender clients cope with reversals in their care plans that may come with age-associated concerns.

Recommended Readings

Ettner, R., Monstrey, S., & Coleman, E. (Eds.). (2016). *Principles of transgender medicine and surgery*. New York, NY: Routledge.

Porter, K. E., Brennan-Ing, M., Chang, S. C., Dickey, L. M., Singh, A. A., Bower, K. L., & Witten, T. M. (2016). Providing competent and affirming services for transgender and gender nonconforming older adults. *Clinical Gerontologist, 39*(5), 366–388.

Wenzel, A., Brown, G. K., & Beck, A. T. (2009). *Cognitive therapy for suicidal patients: Scientific and clinical applications*. Washington, D.C.: American Psychological Association.

References

American Psychiatric Association. (2013). *Diagnostic and statistical manual of mental disorders* (5th edition). Washington, DC: Author.

Asscheman, H., T'Sjoen, G., Lemaire, A., Mas, M., Meriggiola, M. C., Mueller, A., Kuhn, A., Dhejne, C., Morel-Journel, N., & Gooren, L. J. (2014). Venous thrombo-embolism as a complication of cross-sex hormone treatment of male-to-female transsexual subjects: A review. *Andrologia, 46*(7), 791–795.

Beck, A. T., Rush, A. J., Shaw, B. F., & Emery G. (1979). *Cognitive therapy of depression*. New York, NY: Guilford Press.

Beck, J. S. (1995). *Cognitive therapy: Basics and beyond*. New York, NY: Guilford Press.

Baldassarre, M., Giannone, F. A., Foschini, M. P., Battaglia, C., Busacchi, P., Venturoli, S., & Meriggiola, M. C. (2013). Effects of long-term high dose testosterone administration on vaginal epithelium structure and estrogen receptor-α and-β expression of young women. *International Journal of Impotence Research, 25*(5), 172–177.

Bergoglio, M. T., Gómez-Balaguer, M., Folch, E. A., Murillo, F. H., & Hernández-Mijares, A. (2013). Symptomatic meningioma induced by cross-sex hormone treatment in a male-to-female transsexual. *Endocrinologia y Nutricion, 60*(5), 264–267.

Blosnich, J. R., Brown, G. R., Shipherd, J. C., Kauth, M., Piegari, R. I., & Bossarte, R. M. (2013). Prevalence of gender identity disorder and suicide risk among transgender veterans utilizing Veterans Health Administration care. *American Journal of Public Health, 103*(10), e27–e32.

Blosnich, J. R., Brown, G. R., Wojcio, S., Jones, K. T., & Bossarte, R. M. (2014). Mortality among veterans with transgender-related diagnoses in the Veterans Health Administration, FY2000–2009. *LGBT Health, 1*(4), 269–276.

Bockting, W. (2014). The impact of stigma on transgender identity development and mental health. In B. P. C. Kreukels, T. D. Steensma, and A. L.C. deVries (Eds.), *Gender dysphoria and disorders of sex development* (pp. 319–330). New York, NY: Springer.

Bockting, W. O., Miner, M. H., Swinburne-Romine, R. E., Hamilton, A., & Coleman, E. (2013). Stigma, mental health, and resilience in an online sample of the U.S. transgender population. *American Journal of Public Health, 103(5)*, 943–951.

Bowman, E., Oprea, G., Okoli, J., Gundry, K., Rizzo, M., Gabram-Mendola, S., Upender, M., Smith, G., Pambuccian, S., & Bumpers, H. L. (2012). Pseudoangiomatous stromal hyperplasia (PASH) of the breast: A series of 24 patients. *The Breast Journal, 18*(3), 242–247.

Brown, G. R., & Jones, K.T. (2015a). Health correlates of criminal justice involvement in 4,793 transgender veterans. *LGBT Health, 2*(4), 297–305.

Brown, G. R., & Jones, K.T. (2015b). Incidence of breast cancer in a cohort of 5,135 transgender veterans. *Breast cancer research and treatment, 149*(1), 191–198.

Clements-Nolle, K., Marx, R., & Katz, M. (2006). Attempted suicide among transgender persons: The influence of gender-based discrimination and victimization. *Journal of Homosexuality, 51*(3), 53–69.

Cook-Daniels, L. (2016). Understanding transgender elders. In D. A. Harley and P. B. Teaster (Eds.), *Handbook of LGBT elders* (pp. 285–308). New York, NY: Springer International Publishing.

Deipolyi, A. R., Han, S. J., & Parsa, A. T., (2010). Development of a symptomatic intracranial meningioma in a male-to-female transsexual after initiation of hormone therapy. *Journal of Clinical Neuroscience, 17*(10), 1324–1326.

Dhand, A., & Dhaliwal, G. (2010). Examining patient conceptions: A case of metastatic breast cancer in an African American male to female transgender patient. *Journal of General Internal Medicine, 25*(2), 158–161.

Dorff, T. B., Shazer, R. L., Nepomuceno, E. M., & Tucker, S. J. (2007). Successful treatment of metastatic androgen-independent prostate carcinoma in a transsexual patient. *Clinical Genitourinary Cancer, 5*(5), 344–346.

Fredriksen-Goldsen, K. I., Cook-Daniels, L., Kim, H. J., Erosheva, E. A., Emlet, C. A., Hoy-Ellis, C. P., Goldsen, J., & Muraco, A. (2014). Physical and mental health of transgender older adults: An at-risk and underserved population. *The Gerontologist, 54*(3), 488–500.

Ganly, I., & Taylor, E. W. (1995). Breast cancer in a trans-sexual man receiving hormone replacement therapy. *British Journal of Surgery, 82*(3), 341–341.

Gardner, I. H., & Safer, J. D. (2013). Progress on the road to better medical care for transgender patients. *Current Opinion in Endocrinology, Diabetes and Obesity*, *20*(6), 553–558.

Gardner I. H., Safer J. D., Mok S., Weiss R., & Kuohung W. (2014, June). "What is the effect of testosterone on the gene expression in the endometrium of transgender men?" Oral presentation at the World Professional Association for Transgender Health Graduate Student Research Symposium held at the 13th Annual Philadelphia Trans Health Conference, Philadelphia, PA.

Gooren, L., & Morgentaler, A. (2014). Prostate cancer incidence in orchidectomised male-to-female transsexual persons treated with oestrogens. *Andrologia*, *46*(10), 1156–1160.

Gooren, L. J., Giltay, E. J., & Bunck, M. C. (2008). Long-term treatment of transsexuals with cross-sex hormones: Extensive personal experience. *The Journal of Clinical Endocrinology & Metabolism*, *93*(1), 19–25.

Grabellus, F., Worm, K., Willruth, A., Schmitz, K. J., Otterbach, F., Baba, H. A., Kimmig, R. & Metz, K. A. (2005). ETV6–NTRK3 gene fusion in a secretory carcinoma of the breast of a male-to-female transsexual. *The Breast*, *14*(1), 71–74.

Grossman, A. H., & D'Augelli, A. R. (2007). Transgender youth and life-threatening behaviors. *Suicide and Life-Threatening Behavior*, *37*(5), 527–537.

Haas, A. P., Eliason, M., Mays, V. M., Mathy, R. M., Cochran, S. D., D'Augelli, A. R., ... & Russell, S. T. (2011). Suicide and suicide risk in lesbian, gay, bisexual, and transgender populations: Review and recommendations. *Journal of Homosexuality*, *58*(1), 10–51.

Hembree, W. C., Cohen-Kettenis, P., Delemarre-van de Waal, H. A., Gooren, L. J., Meyer, W. J., Spack, N. P., Tangpricha, V., & Montori, V. M. (2009). Endocrine treatment of transsexual persons: An Endocrine Society Clinical Practice Guideline. *Journal of Clinical Endocrinology & Metabolism*, *94*(9), 3132–3154.

Hendricks, M. L., & Testa, R. J. (2012). A conceptual framework for clinical work with transgender and gender nonconforming clients: An adaptation of the Minority Stress Model. *Professional Psychology: Research and Practice*, *43*(5), 460.

Herbst, J. H., Jacobs, E. D., Finlayson, T. J., McKleroy, V. S., Neumann, M. S., Crepaz, N., & HIV/AIDS Prevention Research Synthesis Team. (2008). Estimating HIV prevalence and risk behaviors of transgender persons in the United States: A systematic review. *AIDS and Behavior*, *12*(1), 1–17.

Hughes, T. L., & Eliason, M. (2002). Substance use and abuse in lesbian, gay, bisexual and transgender populations. *Journal of Primary Prevention*, *22*(3), 263–298.

Ikeda, K., Baba, T., Noguchi, H., Nagasawa, K., Endo, T., Kiya, T., & Saito, T. (2012). Excessive androgen exposure in female-to-male transsexual persons of reproductive age induces hyperplasia of the ovarian cortex and stroma but not polycystic ovary morphology. *Human Reproduction*, *28*, 453–461.

Jacobeit, J. W., Gooren, L. J., & Schulte, H. M. (2009). Safety aspects of 36 months of administration of long-acting intramuscular testosterone undecanoate for treatment of female-to-male transgender individuals. *European Journal of Endocrinology*, *161*(5), 795–798.

Jacobson, N. S., Dobson, K. S., Truax, P. A., Addis, M. E., Koerner, K., Gollan, J. K., Gortner, E., & Prince, S. E. (1996). A component analysis of cognitive-behavioral treatment for depression. *Journal of Consulting and Clinical Psychology*, *64*(2), 295.

Jacobson, N. S., Martell, C. R., & Dimidjian, S. (2001). Behavioral activation treatment for depression: Returning to contextual roots. *Clinical Psychology: Science and Practice*, *8*(3), 255–270.

James, S. E., Herman, J. L., Rankin, S., Keisling, M., Mottet, L., & Anafi, M. (2016). *Executive summary of the report of the 2015 U.S. Transgender Survey*. Washington, DC: National Center for Transgender Equality. Retrieved from www.ustranssurvey.org/report/

Kimmel, D. (2014). Lesbian, gay, bisexual, and transgender aging concerns. *Clinical Gerontologist, 37*(1), 49–63.

Kuroda, H., Ohnisi, K., Sakamoto, G., & Itoyama, S. (2008). Clinicopathological study of breast tissue in female-to-male transsexuals. *Surgery Today, 38*(12), 1067–1071.

Lehrman, K. L. (1976). Pulmonary embolism in a transsexual man taking diethylstilbestrol. *JAMA, 235*(5), 532–533.

Linehan, M. M., Comtois, K. A., & Ward-Ciesielski, E. F. (2012). Assessing and managing risk with suicidal individuals. *Cognitive and Behavioral Practice, 19*(2). 218–232.

Luoma, J. B., Kohlenberg, B. S., Hayes, S. C., Bunting, K., & Rye, A. K. (2008). Reducing self-stigma in substance abuse through acceptance and commitment therapy: Model, manual development, and pilot outcomes. *Addiction Research & Theory, 16*(2), 149–165.

Marlatt, G. A. (1996). Harm reduction: Come as you are. *Addictive Behaviors, 21*(6), 779–788.

Marlatt, G. A. & Tapert, S. F. (1993). Harm reduction: Reducing the risks of addictive behaviors. In J. S. Baer, G. A. Marlatt, R. J. McMahon (Eds.), *Addictive behaviors across the life span: Prevention, treatment, and policy issues*. (pp. 243–273). Thousand Oaks, CA: Sage Publications, Inc.

Meyer, W. J., Webb, A., Stuart, C. A., Finkelstein, J. W., Lawrence, B., & Walker, P. A. (1986). Physical and hormonal evaluation of transsexual patients: A longitudinal study. *Archives of Sexual Behavior, 15*(2), 121–138.

Mikhaĭlichenko, V. V., Fesenko, V. N., Khmelnitskiĭ, N. V., Ozhiganova, I. N., Novikov, A. I., Korolev, V. V., & Vasil'ev, V. S. (2013). Morphological and functional changes of organs of female and male reproductive systems at change of sex. *Urologiia (Moscow, Russia: 1999)*, (3), 18–23.

Miller, N., Bedard, Y. C., Cooter, N. B., & Shaul, D. L. (1986). Histological changes in the genital tract in transsexual women following androgen therapy. *Histopathology, 10*(7), 661–669.

Paterson, R. J. (2000). *The assertiveness workbook: How to express your ideas and stand up for yourself at work and in relationships*. Oakland, CA: New Harbinger Publications.

Pattison, S. T., & McLaren, B. R. (2013). Triple negative breast cancer in a male-to-female transsexual. *Internal Medicine Journal, 43*(2), 203–205.

Persson, D. I. (2009). Unique challenges of transgender aging: Implications from the literature. *Journal of Gerontological Social Work, 52*(6), 633–646.

Porter, K. E., Brennan-Ing, M., Chang, S. C., Dickey, L. M., Singh, A. A., Bower, K. L., & Witten, T. M. (2016). Providing competent and affirming services for transgender and gender nonconforming older adults. *Clinical Gerontologist, 39*(5), 366–388.

Pritchard, T. J., Pankowsky, D. A., Crowe, J. P., & Abdul-Karim, F. W. (1988). Breast cancer in a male-to-female transsexual: A case report. *JAMA, 259*(15), 2278–2280.

Reisner, S. L., Pardo, S. T., Gamarel, K. E., Hughto, J. M. W., Pardee, D. J., & Keo-Meier, C. L. (2015). Substance use to cope with stigma in healthcare among US female-to-male trans masculine adults. *LGBT Health, 2*(4), 324–332.

Resmini, E., Andraghetti, G., Rebora, A., Cordera, R., Vera, L., Giusti, M., Minuto, F., & Ferone, D. (2008). Leptin, ghrelin, and adiponectin evaluation in transsexual subjects during hormonal treatments. *Journal of Andrology*, *29*(5), 580–585.

Richmond, K. A., Burnes, T., & Carroll, K. (2012). Lost in trans-lation: Interpreting systems of trauma for transgender clients. *Traumatology*, *18*(1), 45.

Shao, T., Grossbard, M. L., & Klein, P. (2011). Breast cancer in female-to-male transsexuals: two cases with a review of physiology and management. *Clinical Breast Cancer*, *11*(6), 417–419.

Smith, M. J. (1975). *When I say no I feel guilty: How to cope using skills of systemic therapy*. New York, NY: The Daily Press.

Springer, E. (1992). Effective AIDS prevention with active drug users: The harm reduction model. *Journal of Chemical Dependency Treatment*, *4*(2), 141–157.

Stanley, B., & Brown, G. K. (2012). Safety planning intervention: A brief intervention to mitigate suicide risk. *Cognitive and Behavioral Practice*, *19*(2), 256–264.

Symmers, W. S. (1968). Carcinoma of breast in trans-sexual individuals after surgical and hormonal interference with the primary and secondary sex characteristics. *British Medical Journal*, *2*(5597), 83.

Tsemberis, S., Gulcur, L., & Nakae, M. (2004). Housing first, consumer choice, and harm reduction for homeless individuals with a dual diagnosis. *American Journal of Public Health*, *94*(4), 651–656.

Turo, R., Jallad, S., Cross, W. R., & Prescott, S. (2013). Metastatic prostate cancer in transsexual diagnosed after three decades of estrogen therapy. *Canadian Urological Association Journal*, 7(7–8), 544–546.

Urban, R. R., Teng, N. N., & Kapp, D. S. (2011). Gynecologic malignancies in female-to-male transgender patients: The need of original gender surveillance. *American Journal of Obstetrics and Gynecology*, *204*(5), e9–e12.

Weinand, J. D., & Safer, J. D. (2015). Hormone therapy in transgender adults is safe with provider supervision: A review of hormone therapy sequelae for transgender individuals. *Journal of Clinical & Translational Endocrinology*, *2*(2), 55–60.

Wenzel, A., & Beck, A. T. (2008). A cognitive model of suicidal behavior: Theory and treatment. *Applied and Preventive Psychology*, *12*(4), 189–201.

Wenzel, A., Brown, G. K., & Beck, A. T. (2009). *Cognitive therapy for suicidal patients: Scientific and clinical applications*. Washington, DC: American Psychological Association.

Wierckx, K., Elaut, E., Declercq, E., Heylens, G., De Cuypere, G., Taes, Y., Kaufman, J. M., & T'Sjoen, G. (2013). Prevalence of cardiovascular disease and cancer during cross-sex hormone therapy in a large cohort of trans persons: a case–control study. *European Journal of Endocrinology*, *169*(4), 471–478.

Wierckx, K., Elaut, E., Van Hoorde, B., Heylens, G., De Cuypere, G., Monstrey, S., Weyers, S., Hoebeke, P., & T'sjoen, G. (2014). Sexual desire in trans persons: Associations with sex reassignment treatment. *The Journal of Sexual Medicine*, *11*(1), 107–118.

Wierckx, K., Mueller, S., Weyers, S., Van Caenegem, E., Roef, G., Heylens, G., & T'sjoen, G. (2012). Long-term evaluation of cross-sex hormone treatment in transsexual persons. *The Journal of Sexual Medicine*, *9*(10), 2641–2651.

Williams, M. E., & Freeman, P. A. (2007). Transgender health: Implications for aging and caregiving. *Journal of Gay & Lesbian Social Services*, *18*(3–4), 93–108.

Wilson, E. C., Garofalo, R., Harris, R. D., Herrick, A., Martinez, M., Martinez, J., Belzer, M., & The Transgender Advisory Committee and the Adolescent Medicine Trials Network for HIV/AIDS Interventions. (2009). Transgender female youth and sex work: HIV risk and a comparison of life factors related to engagement in sex work. *AIDS Behavior, 13*, 902–913.

Witten, T. M. (2014). It's not all darkness: robustness, resilience, and successful transgender aging. *LGBT Health, 1*(1), 24–33.

World Health Organization. (1993). The ICD-10 classification of mental and behavioural disorders: Diagnostic criteria for research. Retrieved from www.who.int/classifications/icd/en/GRNBOOK.pdf

Yamauchi, T., Kamon, J., Waki, H., Terauchi, Y., Kubota, N., Hara, K., Hara, Y., Mori, T., Ide, K., Murakami, N., Tsuboyama-Kasaoka, O., Ezaki, Y., Akanuma, O., Gavrilova, C., Vinson, M. L., Reitman, H. Kagechika, K., Shudo, M., Yoda, Y., Nakano, K., Tobe, R., Nagai, S., Kimura, M., Tomita, P., & Ezaki, O. (2001). The fat-derived hormone adiponectin reverses insulin resistance associated with both lipoatrophy and obesity. *Nature Medicine*, 7(8), 941–946.

8 Dialectical Behavior Therapy as a Treatment Option for Complex Cases of Gender Dysphoria

Colleen A. Sloan, PhD
Danielle S. Berke, PhD

The views expressed in this material are those of the authors and do not reflect the official policy or position of the Department of Veterans Affairs or the U.S. Government.

Transgender people are at increased risk for mental health concerns (e.g., suicidal ideation, trauma-related distress; for more see Chapter 3). Given the chronic and pervasive invalidation of gender variance within a binary, cisgendered world, some amount of distress about transgender identity can be an expected. This distress may range from non-diagnostic, transient, and mild gender-related distress to extreme and enduring distress affecting functioning across multiple psychosocial domains (e.g., emotion, cognition, behavior), consistent with the DSM-5 diagnosis of Gender Dysphoria (American Psychiatric Association [APA], 2013). For some transgender clients, gender-related distress may be complicated by emotional and behavioral dysregulation, which may develop when best efforts to cope with ongoing invalidation of transgender identity and expression are ineffective. In the absence of learned adaptive coping strategies, a complex clinical picture can emerge. For example, prevalence rates of suicidal ideation and attempts are alarmingly high for transgender individuals (e.g., Blosnich et al., 2013; Blosnich, Brown, Wojcio, Jones, & Bossarte, 2014; Clements-Nolle, Marx, & Katz, 2006; Grossman & D'Augelli, 2007; Haas et al., 2010; Lehavot, Simpson, & Shipherd, 2016) as are rates of risky sexual behavior (Herbst et al., 2008) and substance use (Hughes & Eliason, 2002).

To date, evidence-based approaches to treat Gender Dysphoria that is complicated by emotional and behavioral dysregulation in transgender clients have been quite limited. As such, identification of evidence-based treatment options for complex Gender Dysphoria is an ethical imperative for scholars and mental health professionals alike. This chapter therefore attempts to address this need by describing the application of Dialectical Behavior Therapy (DBT) to the conceptualization and treatment of clients with Gender Dysphoria and associated mental health problems such as suicidality, substance abuse, risky sexual behavior, and other interpersonal challenges (Sloan, Berke, & Shipherd, in press).

DBT is acknowledged as the gold-standard treatment for chronic suicidal behavior and core emotion dysregulation. DBT is based on the premise that clients engage in such behavior in the absence of more adaptive or effective strategies for regulating emotion (Linehan, 1993). As such, DBT targets emotion dysregulation (Lynch, Chapman, Rosenthal, Kuo, & Linehan, 2006). Emotion dysregulation can be defined as the inability to change or regulate emotional cues, experiences, and actions—even when desired and when best efforts are applied (Gross, 2002; 2014). Effective regulation of emotion has been identified as central to mental health and well-being (Gross & Muñoz, 1995). Emotion regulation difficulties, on the other hand, have been associated with a range of maladaptive behaviors including self-harm (Gratz & Roemer, 2004) and substance use (Fox, Axelrod, Paliwal, Sleeper, & Sinha, 2007; Fox, Hong, & Sinha, 2008). Because DBT was designed to target skills deficits, particularly difficulties in emotional and behavioral regulation, the principles and practice of this treatment are highly applicable to the treatment of Gender Dysphoria complicated by comorbidities, such as suicidality, risky sexual behavior, and substance abuse.

DBT is grounded in the Biosocial Model of emotion dysregulation, which describes emotion dysregulation as the consequence of a transactional process between an invalidating environment and biological temperament, marked by emotional vulnerability (Linehan, 1993; 2014). This biological temperament may include characteristics of emotional vulnerability marked by strong emotional reactions to stimuli, which once prompted are high in intensity and long in duration (Crowell, Beauchaine, & Linehan, 2009; Linehan, 1993; 2014). The invalidating environment refers to an environment that fails to acknowledge the validity of an individual's internal experiences including emotions, perceptions, and sense of self.

Within the Biosocial Model, environmental invalidation is posited to transact with biological temperament, giving rise to clinically significant dysregulation of emotion and behavior. By definition, transactional relationship factors simultaneously and continuously influence (i.e., exacerbate) one another over time. Moreover, transactional relationships do not necessarily require equivalency across factors, suggesting that one factor may be considered more severe than the other, but may still result in the same outcome, in this case emotion dysregulation. For some transgender clients, ongoing invalidation of their gender identity may contribute over time to emotion dysregulation and other associated behavioral problems including suicidality, risk-taking, and impulsivity. Emotional and behavioral dysregulation may develop even in the absence of a strong biological vulnerability, due to the severity and pervasiveness of the invalidation to which many transgender individuals are exposed. In fact, even people with very little biological vulnerability may have problems regulating emotion in the context of chronic and pervasive invalidation (Koerner, 2012).

Indeed, transgender individuals are subject to chronic invalidation in a dominant culture that assumes that birth sex and gender identity are interchangeable. Sex assigned at birth is the cultural default for one's gender identity and the binary assumptions of this default are embedded within daily life. For example, many public restrooms and health care clinics are segregated based on biological sex, leaving no clear space for individuals whose gender identity does not conform to sex assigned at birth (Eyler, 2007). This concern is further compounded for people who have non-binary gender identities. Moreover, the social environment actively invalidates transgender identities via institutional discrimination as seen in the absence of discrimination protections for transgender individuals in housing, work settings, and other public sectors in most states across the United States (U.S.; Movement Advancement Project, 2016).

Invalidation of transgender identities and expression in public spaces is evident across cultures. For example, a majority of respondents queried in a series of United Kingdom surveys endorsed receipt of transphobic harassment from strangers in public spaces who perceived them to be transgender (e.g., Morton, 2008; Whittle, Turner, & Al-Alami, 2007). Transgender individuals are also subjected to disproportionate exposure to childhood abuse, intimate partner violence, and violent victimization, relative to their cisgender counterparts (Lombardi, Wilchins, Priesing, & Malouf, 2002; Norton & Herek, 2013; Reisner, White, Bradford, & Mimiaga, 2014; Shipherd, Maguen, Skidmore, & Abramovitz, 2011). In these ways, invalidation is a pervasive component of a transgender individual's environment.

In keeping with the Biosocial Model of emotion dysregulation, transgender individuals are inevitably shaped by their environment. Moreover, an individual's response to the invalidating environment will further influence the environment, exacerbating its invalidating characteristics, which in turn further influence the individual. Over time, this transaction may reasonably impede development of effective emotion regulation strategies (e.g., ability to label, understand, tolerate, modulate, and use emotions to organize effective behavior; Gratz & Roemer, 2004; Linehan, 1993; 2014) and reinforce ineffective emotion regulation strategies (Krause, Mendelson, & Lynch, 2003; Linehan, 1993; 2014) such as suicidal behavior and substance use due to the immediate relief associated with negative reinforcement (alleviation of aversive stimulus).

Transgender individuals whose identity and gender expression are invalidated by the environment may become highly sensitized to the environment's gender-related messages and/or cues and may rely on this environment to shape and "correct" gender non-conforming behavior and expression. They may, for example, seek out activities that promote and reinforce traditional gender roles (e.g., engagement in sports or military culture for transgender women) in an effort to cope with distress engendered by invalidation, thus actively suppressing (self-invalidating) their true gender identity and associated emotions, thoughts, and behavior. Such efforts to suppress true identity are likely ineffective in the long term and may in fact exacerbate emotional distress, as suppression of internal experiences inadvertently increases physiological arousal (Gross, 2002; 2014) and can lead to paradoxical increases in the suppressed experiences (Wegner, 1994). Therefore, transgender clients may evidence vacillation between active self-invalidation/suppression and extreme emotional and behavioral displays as the suppressed content returns. Such behavioral displays may include rigid and/or age inappropriate gendered behavior (e.g., hypermasculine behavior in transgender men), which ultimately functions to regulate the emotional consequences of invalidation. In turn, this extreme behavior elicits further negative responses to transgender identity and expression from the environment. In the absence of effective strategies for managing the effects of a chronically invalidating environment, transgender clients may develop and rely on high-risk behavior including self-harm and substance use in an attempt to communicate distress and/or to self-soothe. Unfortunately, such behavior often has the unintended effect of further disrupting one's ability to establish and maintain affirming social relationships and a stable sense of self.

As the Biosocial Model is the foundation and rationale for DBT, effective application of DBT to the treatment of transgender clients with complex Gender Dysphoria requires that therapists develop an individualized formulation of clients' distress in terms of this model. These formulations are ideally generated in collaboration with the client. Therefore, we recommend providing clients direct feedback about the potential impact of invalidation on their ability to regulate emotions, behavior, and a stable sense of self. The following dialogue illustrates the collaborative refinement of a Biosocial formulation of distress following therapist feedback about diagnostic assessment results:

THERAPIST (T): "What questions do you have about this feedback?"

CLIENT (C): "Well, I guess I don't understand why there's something wrong with me when I'm the one who's dealing with this bigoted world."

T: "I appreciate you being open and honest about your reaction. I apologize if I communicated in any way that something is wrong with you. That was not my intention, and it is not my belief. Rather, I was trying to communicate that emotion dysregulation is the consequence of your chronic experiences of invalidation of your true sense of self. Really, since you were a kid, you've been struggling with these feelings, and you didn't have any kind of outlet to explore them in a healthy way. Right?"

C: "Right, that's true."

T: "So, you stuffed those feelings, which makes sense because you learned that if you didn't, you might be punished."

C: "Yeah, I knew my parents would send me to a looney bin."

T: "Right. So of course you hid them. But you know as well as I do that those feelings didn't go away. And, because you didn't have space to talk about those feelings and manage them, you had more intense feelings to deal with. And because you didn't learn ways to deal with them, you developed many strategies that were not helpful to you in the long run."

C: "I don't get what you mean by 'strategies.'"

T: "When I say strategies, I mean ways of dealing with that underlying distress, the gender dysphoria. In your case, you managed those feelings by suppressing them and engaging in very rigid gender-role behavior, like playing sports, getting into fights."

C: "Sometimes I got into fights because I was just angry. Sometimes I fought to prove I was masculine enough."

T: "Exactly! And that worked, at least temporarily. Then those strategies stopped working, but perhaps leaving you with a hair-trigger reaction to stress, ultimately causing you more distress. And because you never learned to manage that distress effectively, you developed other strategies."

C: "Like drinking and using drugs."

T: "Right. That's how it works. The underlying emotions and difficulties managing those emotions lead to problems in behavior, like fighting and substance use. Then you have even bigger problems to solve. And from what you've told me, these problems also affect your relationships with others."

C: "Yeah, I have real problems with relationships. Part of it is that I have such little support, I'm afraid of losing them so much. But then I end up screwing up and losing them anyway! I don't know what happens!"

T: "Well part of our work together will be to examine that in more detail. We can think about the therapy that we're doing as a 'problem-solving therapy.' You'll be learning skills that are designed to help you solve these problems—change things that aren't working in your life. On the other hand, you'll also be learning skills to help you accept the things that you can't change, at least immediately."

C: "Like what?"

T: "Well, you told me that your parents haven't spoken to you since you came out as transgender, right?"

C: "Right." (becomes tearful)

T: "That's very painful. (pause) Learning to increase acceptance of natural pain is also part of our work. You'll learn more about that in skills training."

The above example also highlights the fundamental dialectic within DBT—acceptance and change. We accept our transgender clients as they are, while simultaneously asking them to makes changes in their lives, namely develop new, effective emotion regulation strategies to replace ineffective behaviors. Within DBT, emotion dysregulation has been described as a "dialectic failure"; that is, a failure to effectively integrate seeming opposites (e.g., emotion and reason/logic). The fundamental dialectic in DBT is that between acceptance and change—therapists accept clients exactly as they are, while simultaneously asking clients to actively work toward behavioral change in the service of improving their lives. The dialectical "dilemma," as applied to transgender individuals struggling with the consequences of invalidation, is the challenge of integrating an affirmed sense of self within an invalidating environment that fails to effectively integrate gender diverse identities. DBT is rooted in dialectical philosophy, a worldview which posits that reality is composed of interrelated parts that cannot be defined without reference to the system as a whole. As applied to psychotherapy, a dialectical philosophy encourages the synthesis of the tension between acceptance and change and a contextual conceptualization of behavior. As such, treatment of complex Gender Dysphoria from a DBT perspective encourages both acceptance of the transgender self within a dominant cisgender world and change strategies to intervene in both the internal self (e.g., self-regulation strategies, physical changes to the body) and the external world (e.g., systems change) to create more validating and affirming space for transgender identities.

DBT prioritizes treatment in such a way as to: 1) keep clients alive by addressing life-threatening behavior; 2) keep clients engaged in treatment by targeting therapy-interfering behavior; and 3) assist clients in developing a life worth living by targeting quality-of-life interfering behavior and other problems (Linehan, 1993; 2014). For example, if a client has recently attempted suicide in the context of significant invalidation of transgender identity (e.g., the client's partner rejects the client and terminates the relationship after the client discloses their transgender identity), a DBT therapist likely would both validate distress associated with such rejection ("It is incredibly painful not to be accepted by someone you love."), while also directly targeting the client's suicidal behavior, with the idea that the client cannot function or proceed successfully in their gender transition if they are actively trying to kill themselves. Likewise, other factors or behavior that pose (potentially imminent) risk and/or interfere with the client's ability to effectively engage in treatment, such as engagement in high-risk sexual behavior, concerning drug use, and homelessness are identified as high priority treatment targets in DBT.

Treatment engagement, as mentioned above, is considered a next priority after life-threatening behavior, and entails collaborative application of problem-solving and skills coaching to promote regular session attendance, homework compliance (e.g., self-monitoring and skill practice), and honest reporting of mutually agreed-upon behavioral targets (e.g., substance use) and internal experiences (i.e., thoughts, emotions, urges). Prioritization of treatment engagement is highly relevant and applicable to work with transgender clients, as transgender individuals experience increased rates of homelessness and poverty (James et al., 2016; Movement Advancement Project, 2016) relative to their cisgender counterparts. Actively acknowledging and collaboratively targeting such barriers as a high priority may increase the accessibility and tolerability of mental health treatment for transgender clients who present with emotional and behavioral dysregulation. Additionally, transgender clients who are habitually confronted with discrimination and/or invalidation (James et al., 2016; Lombardi et al., 2002; Movement Advancement Project, 2016, Norton & Herek, 2013; Reisner,

White, Bradford, & Mimiaga, 2014; Shipherd, Maguen, Skidmore, & Abramovitz, 2011) may be particularly well-served by DBT, given that this treatment approach prioritizes the mutual cultivation of trust and honest communication between client and provider.

Lastly, quality-of-life-interfering behavior and problems include anything that interferes with building a life that is deemed worth living by clients themselves. For transgender clients in particular, Gender Dysphoria can be explicitly targeted here. Herein lies another dialectical dilemma: Gender Dysphoria must be targeted to decrease life-threatening behavior (e.g., suicidality), and life-threatening behavior must cease in order to benefit from interventions to reduce dysphoria. To clarify, this does not necessarily mean that a transgender client cannot gain access to interventions, such as hormone therapy, until they are no longer at risk to themselves (see Chapter 6 for more detail about hormone therapy). Rather, this means that we work collaboratively with clients to keep them alive first, so that they can effectively utilize Gender Dysphoria interventions. Effective utilization of interventions to target Gender Dysphoria may focus on navigating gender transition, selecting relevant interventions, identifying supports, coping with losses, etc. Moreover, any other mental health problems or conditions (e.g., PTSD, problematic substance use) could also be treated/targeted at this level.

As noted earlier, DBT can perhaps be best conceptualized as a "problem-solving therapy" (Linehan, 1993) that embraces a nonjudgmental stance regarding clients' presenting problems. With this in mind, DBT assumes that clients are not to blame or responsible for causing their problems but are indeed responsible for solving them (Linehan, 1993). As applied to work with transgender individuals, this assumption holds that our clients are not responsible for the prejudice, anti-transgender sentiments, or discrimination perpetrated against them, but they are responsible for coping effectively with these experiences, solving their own individual problems, and navigating a gender transition (e.g., taking hormones as prescribed, attending medical appointments, connecting with support) in larger, often unsupportive, contexts.

Below, this problem-solving approach and nonjudgmental stance is modeled by a therapist in dialogue with a client experiencing difficulties gaining access to hormone therapy:

C: "I'm just so sick and tired of having to deal with these stupid rules about what I can and can't do with my own body!"

T: "You're frustrated."

C: Yes, I'm frustrated!"

T: "I get that. Your objective of getting hormone therapy is blocked right now. I'd be frustrated too. At the same time, I'm wondering if we can talk about ways to manage this frustration effectively and use it to help you, not hurt you."

C: "What do you mean?"

T: "Well, remember that the function of frustration is to alert you to problems and help you solve them . . . and to overcome barriers. When your frustration builds and you yell at your endocrinologist, do you think that increases or decreases your chances of getting what you want?"

C: "It decreases it. But I just get so mad!"

T: "Of course you're mad. *And* expressing that anger by yelling gets you further away from your goal of getting hormone therapy. On the other hand, you could use that anger to continue working on smoking cessation, so that you can start hormone treatment."

C: "But that rule is stupid! I've read online that other doctors prescribe hormones even if a person is smoking. Why can't my doctor do that? Quitting smoking is too hard!"

T: "Quitting smoking is hard. There's no arguing that. And you're right that other doctors have different limits. It sounds like working to increase your tolerance of these differences would be helpful at this point, because the reality is that this is your prescriber. Wishing he was different is not actually changing his behavior, right?

C: "Yeah, you're right."

T: "I say this not to say that you shouldn't be upset. I'm not saying that at all. What I am saying is that not accepting that painful reality is only keeping you further from your goal. And I worry that you'll go back to using black market hormones, which we both know is dangerous."

C: "Yes, I know. I've thought about that."

T: "Do you think it's possible that if you were to demonstrate a willingness to even reduce smoking, your endocrinologist might be more willing to start you on hormones?"

C: "Yes, I guess that's a possibility."

T: "Great! Why don't we start there then."

C: "Okay."

For some transgender clients, demonstration and teaching of skills such as problem-solving in an individual mode of therapy is sufficient. For other transgender clients, particularly those who present with severe skills deficits across multiple domains and/or high-risk behavior (e.g., chronic suicidal behavior), full-model, adherent DBT is the recommended treatment approach. Adherent DBT has four modes of treatment including individual psychotherapy, skills training group therapy, telephone consultation, and therapist team consultation, offered with a trained team of providers. The skills training group mode of DBT (Linehan, 1993; 2014) is comprised of four modules: 1) mindfulness, 2) interpersonal effectiveness, 3) distress tolerance, and 4) emotion regulation. Each module functions to target areas of dysregulation: mindfulness to develop a more stable sense of self and address cognitive dysregulation; emotion regulation skills for emotion dysregulation; distress tolerance for behavioral dysregulation; and, interpersonal effectiveness for interpersonal/relationship dysregulation. Overall, the skills training mode balances both change- and acceptance-based strategies. Specifically, mindfulness and distress tolerance are acceptance-based skills, while interpersonal effectiveness and emotion regulation are change-based skills. This balance is key for transgender clients in coping most effectively with the problems identified within this chapter thus far (e.g., substance use, suicidality) and is especially true when transgender clients present with complex Gender Dysphoria.

When considering available interventions for Gender Dysphoria, it is notable that many of these are change-focused (e.g., alterations to one's appearance, hormone therapy, name and gender change, gender confirmation surgeries, voice modulation). While these interventions are likely to alleviate dysphoria, their effectiveness is neither absolute nor assured. For some individuals, these interventions may be too costly, unavailable, or contraindicated by medical conditions.

Gender Dysphoria may also persist following such change-based interventions, particularly in the face of undesired outcomes. For example, some individuals may still be unable to "pass" even after utilizing all available interventions. Additionally, transgender individuals may face ongoing stigma despite considerable investment in change-based interventions. These individual interventions are not designed to create societal change. The limitations of change-focused interventions lead to the other side of the "dialectic"—acceptance. Examples of acceptance-based approaches include support groups (as discussed in Chapter 10) and community building (Chapter 12), which can be useful to bolster clients as they cope with (and potentially advocate for change in) invalidating environments. With this in mind, DBT fosters acquisition of both acceptance and change-based skills to promote optimal adjustment and effective coping. In DBT, clients obtain skills through direct instruction, regular practice, and provision of feedback. Examples of the application of change and acceptance-based skills to treatment when working with transgender clients are provided in Table 8.1.

Table 8.1 Application of dialectical principles and skills to the treatment of complex gender dysphoria

Acceptance		*Change*	
Mindfulness	• Encourage increased contact with a stable sense of self (e.g., attending to true sense of self in larger context of gender-binary environment). • Engage fully in gender affirming activities (e.g., transgender social groups).	Emotion regulation	• Values-based behavior to reduce "hyper" gendered behavior that is inconsistent with identity. • Using problem-solving skills to navigate transition and barriers (e.g., selecting effective interventions; making changes to increase readiness).

(continued)

Table 8.1 Application of dialectical principles and skills to the treatment of complex gender dysphoria *(continued)*

Acceptance		*Change*	
	• Target beliefs about perceived "failures" in gender transition (e.g., "I'm a failure at being a woman if I don't pass"). • Practice loving kindness toward self in context of discrimination. • Mindfulness of others to increase understanding of impact of gender transition and others' difficulties affirming identity (e.g., forgetting name or pronoun).		• Using opposite action to change emotions that interfere with transition and self-affirmation. • Increasing positive social supports and engagement in activities that decrease gender dysphoria. • Building mastery of activities and/or behaviors that are consistent with gender identity. • Coping ahead for anticipated difficulties with transition, discussion of identity with others, potential negative/ disappointing outcomes of intervention.
Distress tolerance/ Reality acceptance	• Acceptance of personal history (e.g., birth sex and given name; experiences as other gender). • History of discrimination. • Acceptance of binary gender system and associated constructions. • Tolerance of slow progress, unexpected outcomes of medical/ physical interventions, lack of availability of services, lack of education (of others). • Learning to sooth self when experiencing pain. • Reducing suffering via acceptance of natural pain associated with marginalized identity and transition.	Interpersonal effectiveness	• Advocating for needs specific to transition (e.g., to providers; requesting support letters). • Advocate for changes in binary gender system; advocate for change in health care policies (e.g., preferred name in system; bathroom access). • Effectively saying "no" to things that increase gender dysphoria (e.g., within relationships). • Requesting others to use preferred name and pronoun. • Establish relationships that affirm gender identity. • Negotiate or end relationships that increase gender dysphoria. • Learn to self-validate true gender identity, particularly in context of invalidation.

It is important to note that the efficacy of DBT has not been explicitly established for the treatment of Gender Dysphoria. As such, the proposal to utilize this approach for both conceptualization and treatment when working with transgender clients who have Gender Dysphoria, particularly when complicated by emotional and behavioral dysregulation, is tentative at this point and based purely on clinical experience and application of theory. Future research should be conducted to evaluate the efficacy of this treatment when working with transgender clients, who may have similar presentations to the population for which DBT was initially developed. Moreover, adherent DBT is quite comprehensive and resource intensive, and its effective implementation requires extensive training. With this in mind, this intervention may not be feasible across all settings. Additionally, the treatment is not recommended, nor can it be identified as effective, if it is not implemented with integrity or not consistent with the model that has been evaluated in the literature (Dimeff & Koerner, 2007).

With the above caveats, DBT is rooted in a solid foundation of evidence-based mental health practices. While DBT was originally developed to treat individuals with chronic and severe suicidal and self-harm behavior, it has since been shown as an effective treatment for other mental health problems including depression (e.g., Linehan et al., 2006), substance use disorders (e.g., Rosenthal, Lynch, & Linehan, 2005), and PTSD (e.g., Harned, Jackson, Comtois, & Linehan, 2010). These data suggest the likely utility of DBT for the treatment of complex Gender Dysphoric clients, as these comorbid diagnoses are overrepresented in the transgender population (Brown & Jones, 2015; Hughes & Eliason, 2002; Shipherd et al., 2011). As such, full-model adherent DBT may be indicated when providing treatment to transgender clients who present with severe dysregulation (e.g., chronic suicidality) and Gender Dysphoria. At a minimum, we recommend skills training for clients presenting with Gender Dysphoria, as improving mindfulness, interpersonal effectiveness, distress tolerance, and emotion regulation skills can be beneficial for many clinical presentations.

Lastly, we argue that the theoretical underpinnings (i.e., Biosocial Model, dialectics) and treatment targets of DBT, including keeping clients alive, engaged in treatment, and effectively working to reduce barriers to high quality of life, are of great applicability to transgender clients, particularly those who present with high-risk behavior. As previously mentioned, transgender individuals are exposed to chronic invalidation within the broader culture (e.g., binary constructs of gender, bathroom laws), environments of care (e.g., clinic waiting rooms, gendered residential treatment facilities), interpersonal encounters (e.g., victimization), and/or in therapeutic contacts (e.g., misgendering, questioning gender identity). Therefore, treatment that targets effective coping with the emotional consequences of these experiences in all relevant contexts is essential for alleviating gender dysphoria and promoting progress in gender transition and overall well-being of transgender clients. Thus, it is recommended that providers flexibly and creatively integrate the general principles and functions of DBT into their work with transgender clients in accordance with their competencies and ethical standards of practice. The following case example is provided to illustrate how a DBT framework may be used to guide the development of an individualized case conceptualization and treatment plan for a transgender client presenting for treatment.

Case Example

CJ is a 24-year old, Caucasian transgender man. For the past four years, he has been dating a cisgender lesbian-identified woman named Karen. They live together in an apartment near CJ's school. He no longer has any relationship with his family of origin. CJ is a full-time college student and is performing well academically, although states that he often feels like he is "holding on by a thread." CJ disclosed his male gender identity to Karen about 2 years ago and notes that their relationship has been strained since that time. CJ describes Karen as supportive, although he also believes that she holds resentment toward his decision to transition. CJ wants Karen to "just play it straight" because her lesbian identity and expression make it harder for him to "pass". CJ has threatened suicide if Karen terminates their relationship and states that he will "do anything" to keep it. Regarding transition goals, CJ desires hormone therapy, legal name and gender marker changes, and gender affirmation surgeries including chest and genital surgeries, although CJ does not believe he will be able to afford either.

CJ currently meets DSM-5 (APA, 2013) criteria for Major Depressive Disorder, Posttraumatic Stress Disorder, Gender Dysphoria, and Tobacco Use Disorder. CJ has a history of suicidal behavior dating back to adolescence. Although CJ describes his suicidal ideation as chronic, occurring "pretty much every day," his history is remarkable for one suicide attempt. When CJ was 15, he "came out" as lesbian and reports that his parents were very unsupportive. He was forced to participate in conversion therapy, which CJ reports led to a suicide attempt via overdose. He also endorses a history of self-harm behavior, marked by hitting himself in the face and head. The frequency of this behavior has fluctuated over time, although it has increased in frequency over the past year. The last instance of this behavior occurred about one week ago in the context of an argument with Karen. CJ also has a history of misusing over-the-counter (OTC) sleep medications to "get a break" from stress.

CJ's history is remarkable for chronic invalidation, as evidenced by his experiences of punishment for his self-identified sexual orientation and gender identity. In fact, his decision to refrain from disclosing gender identity and instead "come out" as a lesbian is indicative of active self-invalidation. Consequently, the Biosocial Model may be a useful framework for conceptualizing his distress. In the context of chronic invalidation, it is likely that CJ learned to suppress his private experiences, which likely affected his ability to trust these experiences, modulate emotions, and communicate needs and wants effectively to others, forcing him to rely on ineffective coping strategies, such as self-harm behavior. These behaviors likely function to regulate negative affect, essentially working to provide temporary relief. Relatedly, CJ attempted suicide on one occasion and experiences chronic suicidal ideation. While further assessment is warranted, it is possible that suicidal and self-harm behavior may unintentionally function to reduce negative affect, gain temporary relief, and communicate distress to others. In particular, CJ's self-harm behavior in the context of interpersonal conflict with partner may function to communicate both how much he values this relationship, as well as communicating his level of distress when confronted with the possibility of losing it. In these ways, suicidal and self-harm behavior may have been inadvertently reinforced (e.g., elicits response from environment), which suggests that CJ has simply learned ineffective coping strategies. This learning has likely contributed to specific difficulties in coping with Gender Dysphoria, which in turn is exacerbated by ongoing experiences of invalidation.

Considering the hierarchy of treatment targets, a DBT approach would first target life-threatening behavior, obtaining commitment from CJ to stay alive, reduce suicidal behavior (including verbalization without intent), reduce self-harm behavior, and reduce misuse of OTC sleep medications, which is a risk factor for accidental overdose and death. Secondly, any therapy-interfering behavior should be targeted including attendance, completion of self-monitoring forms (i.e., diary cards), and regular practice of skills. Lastly, quality-of-life-interfering behavior and issues are targeted, most importantly, Gender Dysphoria and active engagement in behavior toward transition-related goals. Focusing on the aforementioned prioritized targets (e.g., suicidal behavior) will allow for more effective utilization of interventions and coping with Gender Dysphoria. Additionally, other mental health concerns, including PTSD, depression, and relationship problems, are treated within a quality-of-life intervention level.

Regarding skills practice, it likely will be important to emphasize use of distress tolerance and other acceptance skills to increase acceptance of painful realties (e.g., non-affirmation of his gender identity from loved ones, discriminatory legislation against transgender people) as well as skills to tolerate distress and manage crises without engaging in suicidal, self-harm, or impulsive behavior that makes crisis situations worse. Likewise, mindfulness skills can help CJ increase awareness of internal experiences, nonjudgmentally, and encourage balanced thinking and decision-making, as well as a stable sense of self. Change-focused skills include interpersonal effectiveness, which aims to target CJ's ineffective interpersonal behavior. These skills can aid CJ in effectively communicating with his partner as well as health care professionals, particularly when he begins pursuing hormone therapy, and perhaps eventually gender confirmation surgeries. Moreover, the interpersonal skills module includes content that promotes recovery from interpersonal invalidation, which likely would benefit CJ, particularly within his relationship. It will be important to discuss ways to encourage validation of both CJ and Karen, as CJ's decision to transition differentially impacts each of them. Emotion regulation skills can assist CJ, in general, with more effectively managing emotions and using them to guide engagement in goal-oriented behavior (e.g., studying for exams, contacting and choosing a hormone therapy provider). Generally, a balance of acceptance- and change-based interventions (as the fundamental dialectic in DBT) will be important.

As CJ begins to progress in his gender transition, this affects his relationship with a cisgender, lesbian-identified woman. While CJ has a strong desire to maintain this relationship, his gender identity as a man may be invalidated within this relationship, as his partner is attracted to women and self-identifies as a lesbian. It may be possible to reconcile these dilemmas and promote effective gender transition while maintaining this relationship. At the same time, given that loss or change in this relationship is possible, skills training should focus on effective coping and self-validation without relying on suicidal or self-harm behavior.

Take Home Points

- Transgender clients are at increased risk for several mental health conditions.
- Although gender-related distress is an expected consequence of chronic and pervasive invalidation of transgender identity, it may be accompanied and exacerbated by underlying emotion and behavior dysregulation.
- DBT is an effective treatment for emotion dysregulation and identity development; as such, the underlying Biosocial Model informs conceptualization of gender-related distress and complex Gender Dysphoria.
- DBT may be a treatment option for Gender Dysphoria when the client's presentation is complicated by emotion and behavioral dysregulation.
- DBT skills training can increase effective coping with invalidation, by decreasing emotion and behavior dysregulation.

Recommended Readings

Koerner, K. (2012). *Doing dialectical behavior therapy: A practical guide*. New York, NY: Guilford Press.

Linehan, M. M. (1993). *Cognitive-behavioral treatment of borderline personality disorder*. New York, NY: Guilford Press.

Linehan, M. M. (2014). *DBT® skills training manual*. New York, NY: Guilford Press.

For training opportunities: http://behavioraltech.org/index.cfm

References

American Psychiatric Association. (2013). *Diagnostic and statistical manual of mental disorders* (5th edition). Washington, DC: Author.

Blosnich, J. R., Brown, G. R., Shipherd, J. C., Kauth, M., Piegari, R. I., & Bossarte, R. M. (2013). Prevalence of gender identity disorder and suicide risk among transgender veterans utilizing Veterans Health Administration care. *American Journal of Public Health, 103*, e27–e32.

Blosnich, J. R., Brown, G. R., Wojcio, S., Jones, K. T., & Bossarte, R. M. (2014). Mortality among veterans with transgender-related diagnoses in the Veterans Health Administration, FY2000–2009. *LGBT Health, 1*(4), 269–276.

Brown, G. R., & Jones, K. T. (2015). Mental health and medical health disparities in 5135 transgender veterans receiving healthcare in the Veterans Health Administration: A case–control study. *LGBT Health, 3*, 122–131.

Clements-Nolle, K., Marx, R., & Katz, M. (2006). Attempted suicide among transgender persons: The influence of gender-based discrimination and victimization. *Journal of Homosexuality, 51*, 53–69.

Crowell, S. E., Beauchaine, T. P., & Linehan, M. M. (2009). A biosocial developmental model of borderline personality disorder: Elaborating and extending Linehan's theory. *Psychological Bulletin, 135*, 495–510.

Dimeff, L. A., & Koerner, K. E. (2007). *Dialectical behavior therapy in clinical practice: Applications across disorders and settings.* New York, NY: Guilford Press.

Eyler, A. E. (2007). Primary medical care of the gender-variant patient. In R. Ettner, S. Monstrey, & A. E. Eyler (Eds.), *Principles of transgender medicine and surgery* (pp. 15–32). New York, NY: The Haworth Press.

Fox, H. C., Axelrod, S. R., Paliwal, P., Sleeper, J., & Sinha, R. (2007). Difficulties in emotion regulation and impulse control during cocaine abstinence. *Drug and Alcohol Dependence, 89*(2), 298–301.

Fox, H. C., Hong, K. A., & Sinha, R. (2008). Difficulties in emotion regulation and impulse control in recently abstinent alcoholics compared with social drinkers. *Addictive Behaviors, 33*(2), 388–394.

Gratz, K. L., & Roemer, L. (2004). Multidimensional assessment of emotion regulation and dysregulation: Development, factor structure, and initial validation of the difficulties in emotion regulation scale. *Journal of Psychopathology and Behavioral Assessment, 26*, 41–54.

Gross, J. J. (2002). Emotion regulation: Affective, cognitive, and social consequences. *Psychophysiology, 39*, 281–291.

Gross, J. J. (2014). *Handbook of emotion regulation.* (2nd ed.). New York, NY: The Guilford Press.

Gross, J. J., & Muñoz, R. F. (1995). Emotion regulation and mental health. *Clinical psychology: Science and Practice, 2*(2), 151–164.

Grossman, A. H., & D'Augelli, A. R. (2007). Transgender youth and life-threatening behaviors. *Suicide and Life-Threatening Behavior, 37*, 527–537.

Haas, A. P., Eliason, M., Mays, V. M., Mathy, R. M., Cochran, S. D., D'Augelli, A. R., Silverman, M. M., Fisher, P. W., Hughes, T., Rosario, M., Russell, S. T., Malley, E., Reed, J., Litts, D. A., Haller, E., Sell, R. L., Remafedi, G., Bradford, J., Beautrais, A. L., Brown, G. K., Diamond, G. M., Friedman, M. S., Garofalo, R., Turner, M. S., Hollibaugh, A., & Clayton, P. J. (2010). Suicide and suicide risk in lesbian, gay, bisexual, and transgender populations: review and recommendations. *Journal of Homosexuality, 58*, 10–51.

Harned, M. S., Jackson, S. C., Comtois, K. A., & Linehan, M. M. (2010). Dialectical behavior therapy as a precursor to PTSD treatment for suicidal and/or self-injuring women with borderline personality disorder. *Journal of Traumatic Stress, 23*, 421–429.

Herbst, J. H., Jacobs, E. D., Finlayson, T. J., McKleroy, V. S., Neumann, M. S., Crepaz, N., & HIV/AIDS Prevention Research Synthesis Team. (2008). Estimating HIV prevalence and risk behaviors of transgender persons in the United States: A systematic review. *AIDS and Behavior, 12*, 1–17.

Hughes, T. L., & Eliason, M. (2002). Substance use and abuse in lesbian, gay, bisexual and transgender populations. *Journal of Primary Prevention, 22*, 263–298.

James, S. E., Herman, J. L., Rankin, S., Keisling, M., Mottet, L., & Anafi, M. A. (2016). *The report of the 2015 US Transgender Survey.* Washington: National Center for Transgender Equality. Retrieved from www.transequality.org/sites/default/files/docs/usts/USTS%20Full%20Report%20-%20FINAL%201.6.17.pdf

Koerner, K. (2012). *Doing dialectical behavior therapy: A practical guide.* New York, NY: Guilford Press.

Krause, E. D., Mendelson, T., & Lynch, T. R. (2003). Childhood emotional invalidation and adult psychological distress: The mediating role of emotional inhibition. *Child Abuse & Neglect, 27*, 199–213.

Lehavot, K., Simpson, T.L., & Shipherd, J.C. (2016). Factors associated with suicidality among a national sample of transgender veterans. *Suicide and Life Threatening Behavior, 46*(5), 507–524.

Linehan, M. M. (1993). *Cognitive-behavioral treatment of borderline personality disorder.* New York, NY: Guilford Press.

Linehan, M. M. (2014). *DBT® skills training manual.* New York, NY: Guilford Press.

Linehan, M. M., Comtois, K. A., Murray, A. M., Brown, M. Z., Gallop, R. J., Heard, H. L., Korslund, K. E., Tutek, D. A., Reynolds, S.K., & Lindenboim, N. (2006). Two-year randomized controlled trial and follow-up of dialectical behavior therapy vs therapy by experts for suicidal behaviors and borderline personality disorder. *Archives of General Psychiatry, 63*, 757–766.

Lombardi, E. L., Wilchins, R. A., Priesing, D., & Malouf, D. (2002). Gender violence: Transgender experiences with violence and discrimination. *Journal of Homosexuality, 42*, 89–101.

Lynch, T. R., Chapman, A. L., Rosenthal, M. Z., Kuo, J. R., & Linehan, M. M. (2006). Mechanisms of change in dialectical behavior therapy: Theoretical and empirical observations. *Journal of Clinical Psychology, 62*, 459–480.

Morton, J. (2008). *Transgender Experiences in Scotland: Research Summary. Scottish Transgender Alliance.* Retrieved from www.scottishtrans.org/wp-content/uploads/2013/03/staexperiencessummary03082.pdf

Movement Advancement Project (2016). *State Non-Discrimination Laws [map].* Retrieved from www.lgbtmap.org/equality-maps/non_discrimination_laws

Norton, A. T., & Herek, G. M. (2013). Heterosexuals' attitudes toward transgender people: Findings from a national probability sample of US adults. *Sex Roles, 68*, 738–753.

Reisner, S. L., White, J. M., Bradford, J. B., & Mimiaga, M. J. (2014). Transgender health disparities: Comparing full cohort and nested matched-pair study designs in a community health center. *LGBT Health, 1*, 177–184.

Rosenthal, M. Z., Lynch, T. R., & Linehan, M. M. (2005). Dialectical behavior therapy for individuals with borderline personality disorder and substance use disorders.

In R. J. Frances, S. I. Miller, & A. H. Mack (Eds.), *Clinical textbook of addictive disorders*, 615–636. New York, NY: The Guilford Press.

Shipherd, J. C., Maguen, S., Skidmore, W. C., & Abramovitz, S. M. (2011). Potentially traumatic events in a transgender sample: Frequency and associated symptoms. *Traumatology*, *17*, 56–67.

Sloan, C. A., Berke, D. S., & Shipherd, J. C. (in press). Utilizing a dialectical framework to inform conceptualization and treatment of clinical distress in transgender individuals. *Professional Psychology Research and Practice.*

Wegner, D. M. (1994). Ironic processes of mental control. *Psychological Review*, *101*, 34–52.

Whittle, S., Turner, L., & Al-Alami, M. (2007). *Engendered penalties: Transgender and transsexual people's experiences of inequality and discrimination*. London: The Equalities Review.

9 Pursuing Gender Transitioning Surgeries

Loren S. Schechter, MD
Rebecca B. Schechter, MD

For individuals pursuing surgery, medical and mental health professionals can review the spectrum of available procedures, provide presurgical evaluations, discuss the timing of surgical interventions, help the individual understand the support required in the postoperative period, and assist with postsurgical care. In this chapter, we discuss the surgeon's role in the interdisciplinary team, the preoperative evaluation for surgery, the variety of available surgical options, and the postoperative care. In addition, we address the rapidly evolving health care environment, with specific attention to improving access and recognizing ongoing barriers faced by this underserved population.

Appropriate Candidates for Gender Affirming Surgery

Not all persons with gender dysphoria desire surgery. The decision to pursue a surgical intervention is personal and requires individualized care. In those individuals who request surgery, the extent of surgical interventions may vary. In this regard, the mental health professional plays a central role in helping individuals identify therapeutic interventions that may be of benefit. Because surgery is irreversible, the World Professional Association for Transgender Health (WPATH) *Standards of Care (SOC)* guidelines recommend "persistent, well-documented gender dysphoria" as a criterion for all chest and genital surgery (WPATH *SOC*, 2011). In addition, for some procedures, hormone therapy and one year of continuous living in the gender role congruent with one's gender identity is recommended. It is important to recognize that the *SOC* were not developed as a barrier to care, but as guidelines, designed to help provide appropriate care. This concept is especially important when considering surgery.

The *SOC* recommends written referral letters from mental health providers in order to document that an individual has undergone an assessment for surgery. The number of evaluations/referral letters depends upon the particular surgery. In general, chest/breast surgery requires one referral letter, whereas genital surgery requires two letters. Per the *SOC* (WPATH, 2011), referral letters should include:

1. The client's general identifying characteristics;
2. Results of the client's psychosocial assessment, including any diagnoses;
3. The duration of the mental health professional's relationship with the client, including the type of evaluation and therapy or counseling to date;
4. An explanation that the criteria for surgery have been met, and a brief description of the clinical rationale for supporting the patient's request for surgery;
5. A statement about the fact that informed consent has been obtained from the patient;
6. A statement that the mental health professional is available for coordination of care and welcomes a phone call to establish this.

In addition to these referral letters, an evaluation from an individual's primary care provider or endocrinologist, when indicated, may assist with preoperative preparation of the patient.

The Role of the Surgeon in the Health Care Team

The surgeon should take an active role in the interdisciplinary health care team. As such, communication between health care providers is essential in optimizing the treatment plan. It is important for the surgeon to understand the individual's diagnosis as well as the appropriateness of surgical therapy. Communication with mental health providers also helps the surgeon understand the particular needs of the individual. Finally, it is the responsibility of the surgeon to communicate pertinent operative findings as well as postoperative instructions with the health care team (Schechter, 2009).

Preoperative Evaluation

An in-person preoperative surgical consultation is required. During this visit the procedure(s) and postoperative course are described, the potential risks and benefits of surgery are reviewed, and the individual's questions are answered. The surgeon must also learn about the individual's expectations and explain the limitations of surgery. Individuals who have unrealistic expectations risk disappointment in their final results.

The surgeon must also consider an individual's comorbid mental health and medical problems that may affect surgery and postoperative care. Mental health and primary care providers should work to ensure that these conditions are managed prior to the intervention, and that the individual is optimized for surgery.

Certain conditions, especially obesity and smoking, can adversely affect surgical outcomes and should also be addressed before surgery. In the lead author's opinion, a body mass index (BMI) greater than 30 can increase the risk of complications and, especially in genital surgery, result in poor aesthetic and functional results. As such, weight loss should be encouraged prior to surgery. Smoking can result in delayed healing and necrosis of grafts and flaps. It is the lead author's practice to have individuals discontinue smoking at least six weeks prior to surgery. Compliance can be confirmed with measurement of urine cotinine, and surgery may be postponed based upon the test results.

If an individual decides to proceed with surgery, written documentation of informed consent should be included in the patient's chart.

Gender Affirming Surgeries

Feminizing Genital Surgery

Vaginoplasty, or creation of a neovagina, is the mainstay of feminizing genital surgery. Vaginoplasty techniques were originally developed for the treatment of vaginal agenesis (not fully formed or developed vaginas) (McIndoe & Bannister, 1938) and have been adapted to serve the needs of transgender women. Functional vaginoplasty can be performed in a single operation. However, some individuals choose to undergo an additional labiaplasty as a secondary procedure. This secondary labiaplasty is less common as, nowadays, many women perform hair removal of the mons region. As such, they prefer to forego the additional incisions in the mons area.

There are three surgical options for vaginoplasty: penile inversion vaginoplasty, intestinal transplantation, or nongenital flaps. Most centers perform primary vaginoplasty with the penile inversion technique; this technique uses penile skin combined with scrotal-perineal tissue and/or skin grafts to create a neovagina. Intestinal vaginoplasty, which uses vascularized colonic or ileal segments to create a vagina with a moist lining, is typically reserved for revision cases in which there has been vaginal stenosis (narrowing of the opening). The advantage of intestinal transposition is the creation of a vascularized 12–15 cm vagina with a moist lining. This may lessen the requirements for postoperative vaginal dilation as well as the need for lubrication during intercourse. However, the drawbacks of intestinal transposition include the need for an intra-abdominal operation with a bowel anastomosis (surgical connection of distinct structures) and the potential for neovaginal secretions. Intestinal vaginoplasty may become more commonplace as adolescents undergo pubertal suppression. Pubertal suppression may result in penoscrotal hypoplasia (incomplete development) and insufficient tissue for a penile inversion vaginoplasty. Non-genital flaps are typically considered for reconstruction following oncologic resections.

Regardless of the technique utilized, hormones are discontinued approximately two weeks prior to surgery in order to reduce the risk of venous thromboembolism (VTE), and a preoperative bowel preparation is administered the day prior to surgery.

Penile Inversion Vaginoplasty

Hair removal, whether by electrolysis or laser, is completed as thoroughly as possible from the penile shaft, central perineum, and scrotum prior to penile inversion vaginoplasty. This helps prevent hair growth in the neovagina. Adequate hair removal can take several months to complete and should not be performed within 2 weeks of surgery.

Although several technical modifications are utilized in the penile inversion vaginoplasty, the component parts of the penis are disassembled, and the skin is inverted and combined with a posteriorly-based, scrotal-perineal flap to form the vaginal cavity. (See Figure 9.1.) The labia majora are formed from the lateral remnants of the scrotum, the neoclitoris is formed from the dorsal glans penis, and the labia minora are formed from the penile skin and a urethral flap. The penile urethra is shortened and spatulated (enlarged at the end) to create the neourethral opening and vestibular lining. Depending upon the length of the penis and previous circumcision, skin grafts may be required for additional vaginal depth.

The postoperative care consists of a variable period of bed rest, during which a vaginal stent or packing is used to maintain the vaginal cavity. Once the vaginal stent is removed, a regimen of vaginal dilation with a prosthesis

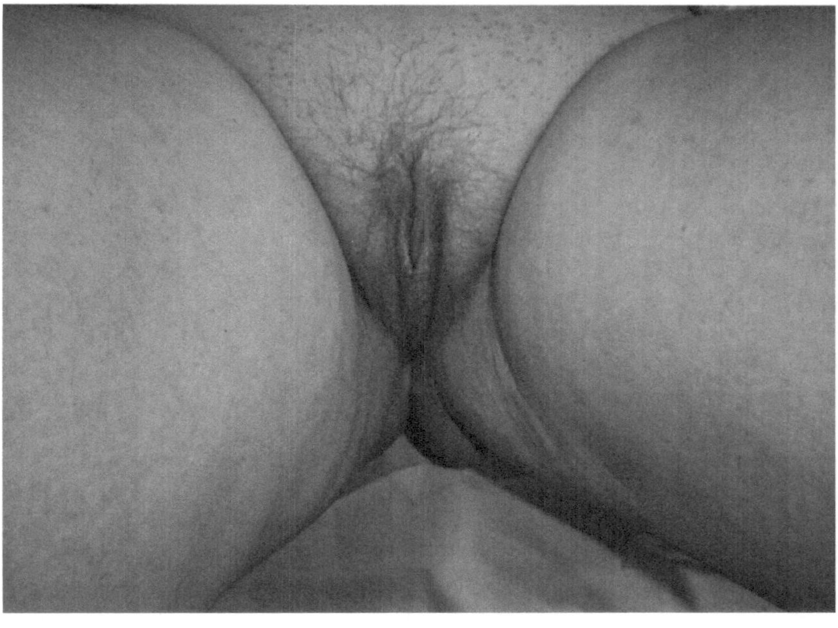

Figure 9.1 Postoperative penile inversion vaginoplasty (photo used with permission of subject)

is initiated. Additionally, intermittent vaginal douching with a diluted povidine-iodine solution is performed to remove intravaginal debris. Vaginal intercourse may begin 6 to 8 weeks after surgery.

Protocols for vaginal dilation may vary based upon individual circumstances and the surgeon's preference. Either vaginal dilation or vaginal intercourse is required on a lifelong basis. Typical dilation regimens decrease over time.

Early postoperative complications include bleeding, infection, and delayed wound healing. Other complications include rectovaginal fistula (abnormal opening), urinary stream abnormalities, inadequate vaginal depth or a constricted introitus (entrance of the cavity), partial flap loss, loss of neoclitoral sensation, and an unsatisfactory cosmetic appearance.

Intestinal Vaginoplasty

The advantage of intestinal transposition is the provision of a reliable length of vascularized tissue with mucus secretion providing lubrication for vaginal intercourse. The sigmoid colon is most commonly used for intestinal transposition due to its larger luminal (tubular) diameter and less copious secretions compared to the jejunum or ileum. Prior to performing the sigmoid vaginoplasty, a preoperative colonoscopy is performed to evaluate for pre-existing colorectal malignancies.

The sigmoid vaginoplasty (see Figure 9.2) is performed in conjunction with general surgery. A combined abdominal and perineal approach is utilized. This allows visualization and protection of the bladder and urethra anteriorly and the rectum posteriorly. The sigmoid colon is harvested by the general surgery team, often with laparoscopic assistance, while the plastic surgery team performs the perineal dissection. The low pelvic dissection may be assisted with the use of the operating robot. A 12–15 cm segment of sigmoid colon is transferred and sutured to the introitus of the neovagina. The mesentery (membranous fold of tissue) of the defunctionalized sigmoid colon may be sewn to the pelvis to prevent torsion. An end-to-end colonic anastomosis is performed to restore intestinal continuity, and the distal stump of the neovagina is separated from the colonic anastomosis.

The neovagina is packed with non-adherent gauze, and the patient remains on bed rest with a urinary catheter for 1 to 2 days. Upon return of bowel function and oral intake, the patient is discharged from the hospital.

The potential drawbacks of intestinal-based flaps include secretions, most notably with the small intestine, and possible malodorous discharge with the large intestine. Additional concerns include the possibility of diversion colitis (inflammation of the nonfunctioning pouch) in the defunctionalized sigmoid colon, as well as the risk of gastrointestinal malignancies. Finally, the colonic mucosa may be somewhat friable (crumbly or brittle), and small amounts of post-coital bleeding may occur.

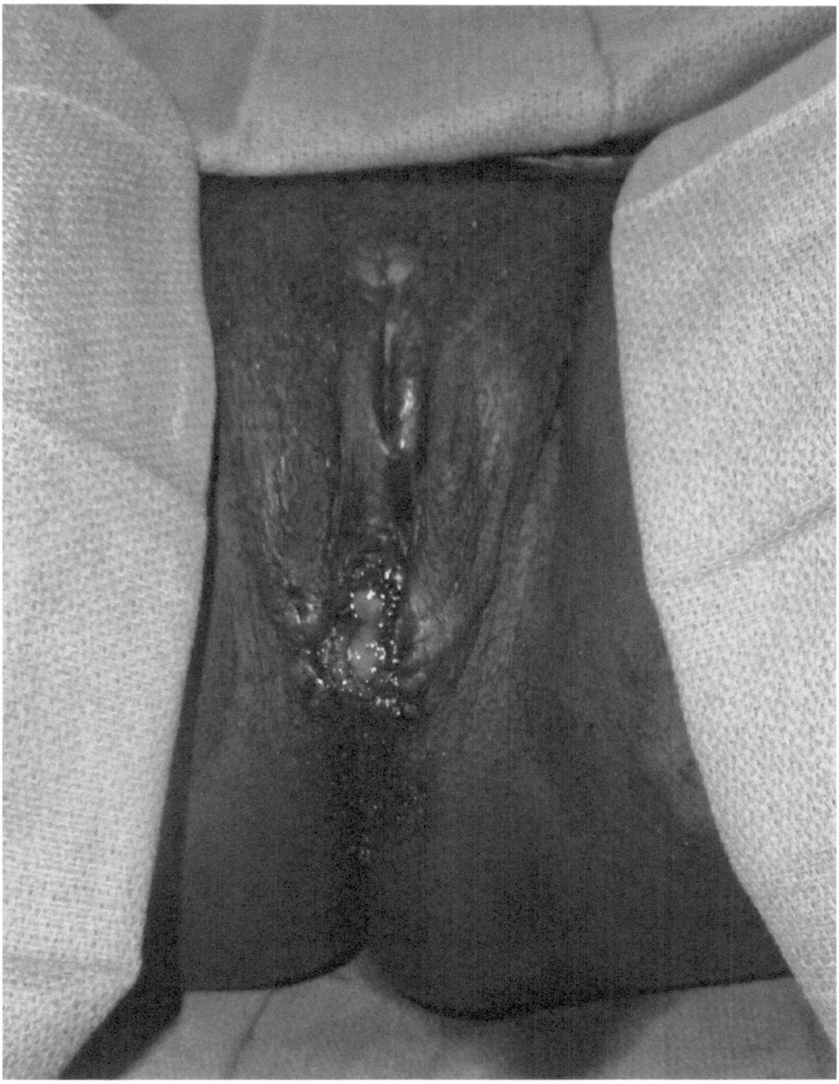

Figure 9.2 Postoperative intestinal vaginoplasty (photo used with permission of subject)

Feminizing Chest Surgery and Facial Feminization

Additional feminizing procedures include both chest surgery and facial feminization. The goal of these procedures is to remove the secondary sexual characteristics associated with the stereotypic male appearance. The timing of these surgeries in relation to genital surgery is variable and depends on the individual's goals of therapy. These feminizing procedures are commonly performed prior to genital surgery to improve the individual's sense of well-being (Monstrey et al., 2001).

Following hormonal therapy, there is often some breast growth in transgender women. However, the breast growth is often inadequate, and many individuals continue to wear external prostheses or padded bras. As such, breast augmentation may be requested. Anatomic differences between the male and female chest are relevant as to implant selection, incision choice, and pocket location (Kanhai, Hage, Bloemena, van Diest, & Karim, 1999).

The male chest is wider than the female chest, and the pectoralis major muscle is usually more developed. Furthermore, the male areola is smaller than the female areola, the distance between the nipple and the inframammary crease is shorter, and there is less ptosis (sagging) in the transgender woman's breast, even after hormonal therapy (Laub, 1999). For these reasons, a larger implant is commonly chosen. (See Figures 9.3a and 9.3b.) Pocket location and incision choice depend upon individual characteristics. Most often, silicone implants and, more recently, form-stable silicone implants are utilized.

In addition to breast augmentation, surgery to feminize the face may be requested. A variety of characteristics associated with the forehead, nose, malar (cheek) region, mandible, and thyroid cartilage are often identified as masculine.

Because the female eyebrow is located higher and has a more arched appearance than the male, a brow lift with advancement of the frontal hairline and frontal bone reduction can be performed. Depending upon the amount of frontal bone thickness, other craniofacial surgical techniques may be required to achieve the desired appearance.

A feminizing rhinoplasty typically involves nasal bridge reshaping, nasal tip trimming and elevation, and narrowing of the nasal pyramid. (See Figures 9.4a and 9.4b.) Individuals may also request feminization of the chin and mandible. Based upon the individual's anatomy, either chin implants or chin reshaping may be required. In addition, reduction of the masseter muscle and/or jaw bone may be performed through intraoral incisions. Other procedures, such as upper lip shortening, facelift, blepharoplasty (eyelid lift), malar implants, hair transplantation, injectable fillers, and skin resurfacing may also be performed.

Reduction thyroid chondroplasty ("tracheal shave") may be requested to reduce the appearance of the "Adam's apple" or prominent thyroid cartilage. (See Figures 9.5a and 9.5b.) This procedure is typically performed as an outpatient, under general or local anesthesia with sedation. The procedure is performed through a transverse incision in a naturally occurring neck skin crease.

Voice surgery, designed to raise vocal pitch, may be requested. (See Chapter 10 on Adjunctive Interventions for more information). Hormonal intervention does not commonly affect vocal pitch, and many individuals are bothered by this residual stigma of masculinity. As such, various techniques

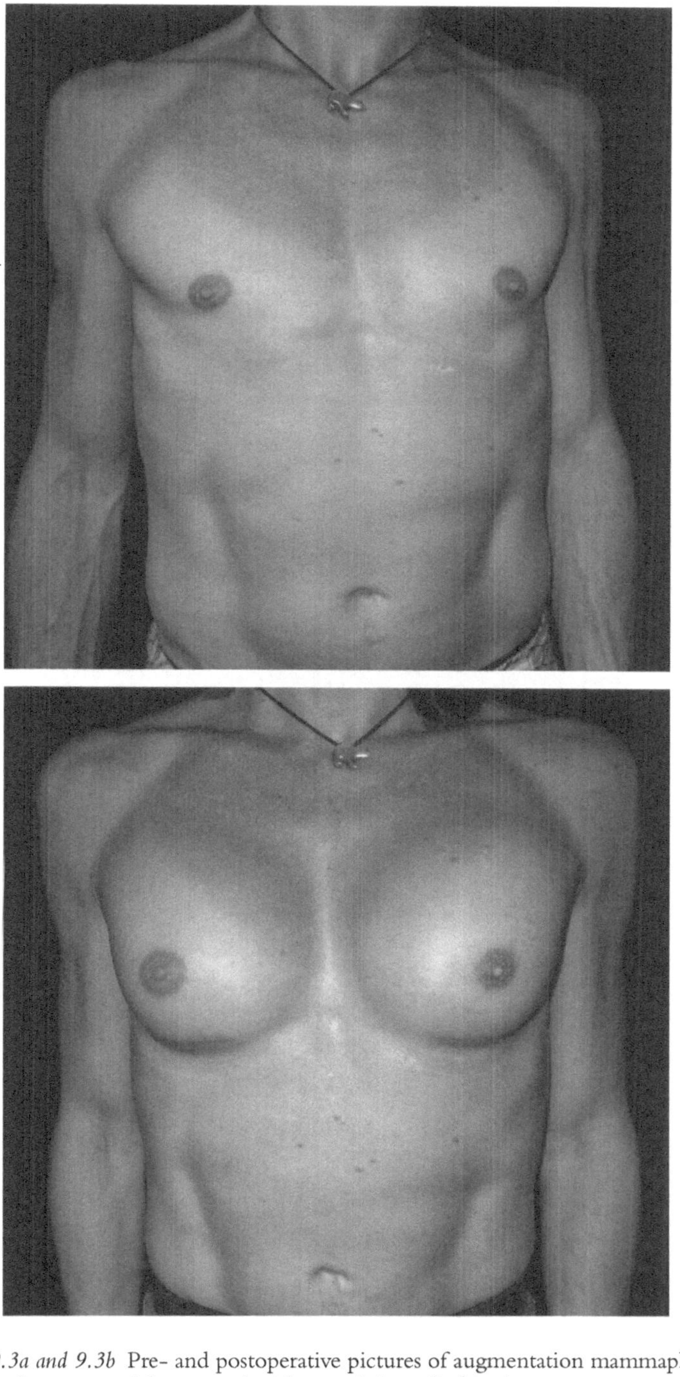

Figures 9.3a and 9.3b Pre- and postoperative pictures of augmentation mammaplasty in a transgender woman (photos used with permission of subject)

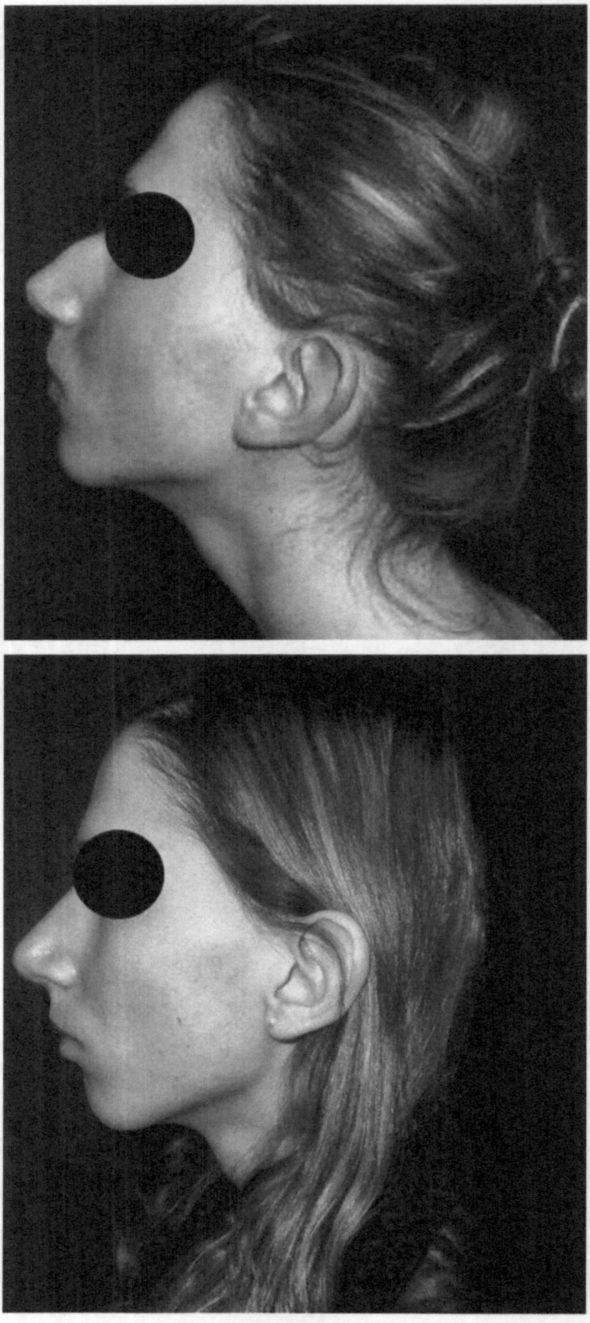

Figures 9.4a and 9.4b Pre- and postoperative pictures of rhinoplasty (photos used with permission of subject)

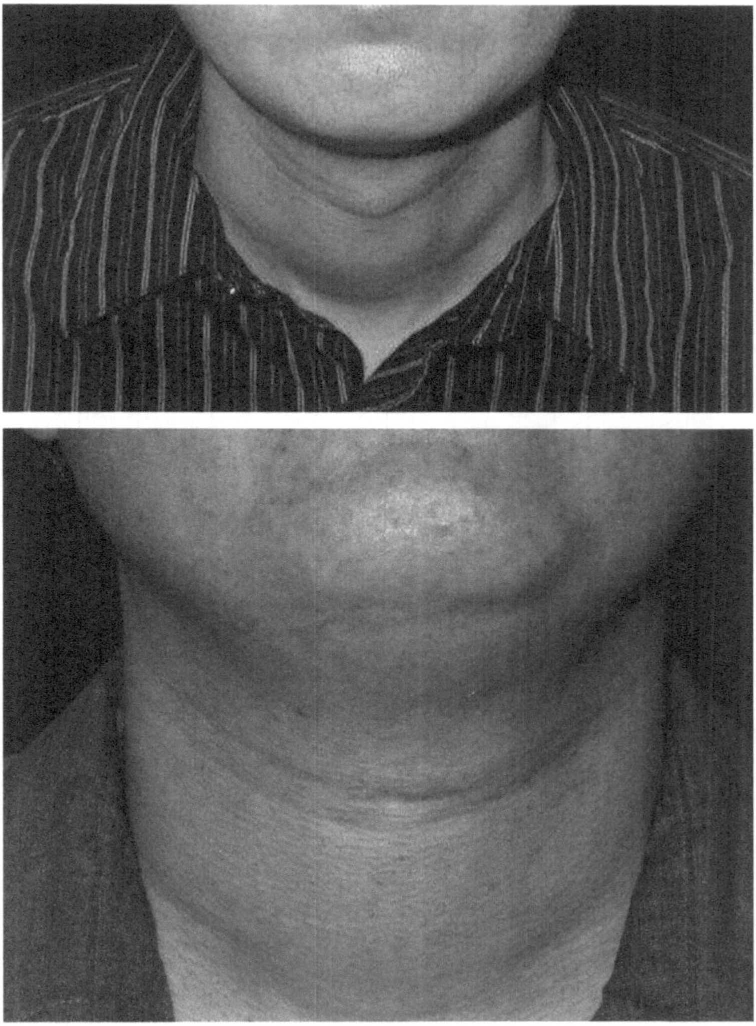

Figures 9.5a and 9.5b Pre- and postoperative pictures of tracheal shave in a transgender woman (photos used with permission of subject)

to shorten the vocal cords, increase vocal cord tension, or reduce vibrating vocal cord mass may be performed (Ettner, 2007), although the efficacy of such surgeries is uncertain (Lechien et al., 2014; McNeill, 2006).

Masculinizing Chest Surgery

Chest-wall contouring is an important early surgical step in the process of gender confirmation for transgender men. The goals of masculinizing chest surgery include the aesthetic contouring of the chest by removal of breast tissue and skin excess, reduction and repositioning of the nipple-areola complex, release of the inframammary crease (the area where the lower edge of the breast meets the chest wall), and minimization of chest scars (Monstrey et al., 2008).

There are several techniques employed in performing masculinizing chest surgery. These are related to breast volume, breast ptosis, nipple-areola size and position, degree of skin excess, and potential loss of skin elasticity, often related to long-term breast binding. (See Figures 9.6a and 9.6b.) Choice of

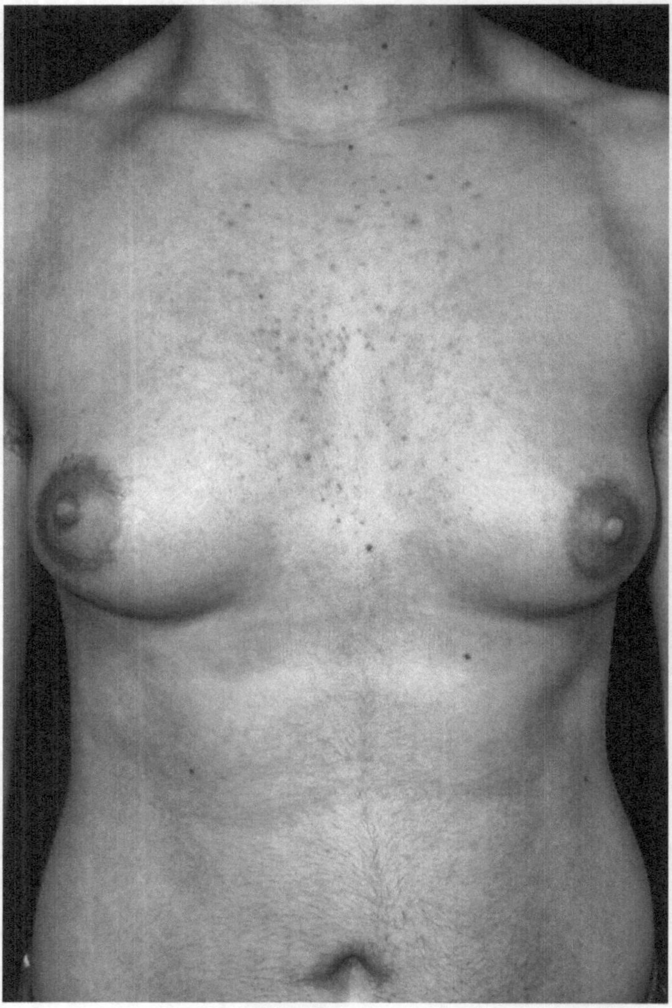

Figures 9.6a and 9.6b Pre- and postoperative masculinizing chest surgery (photos used with permission of subject)

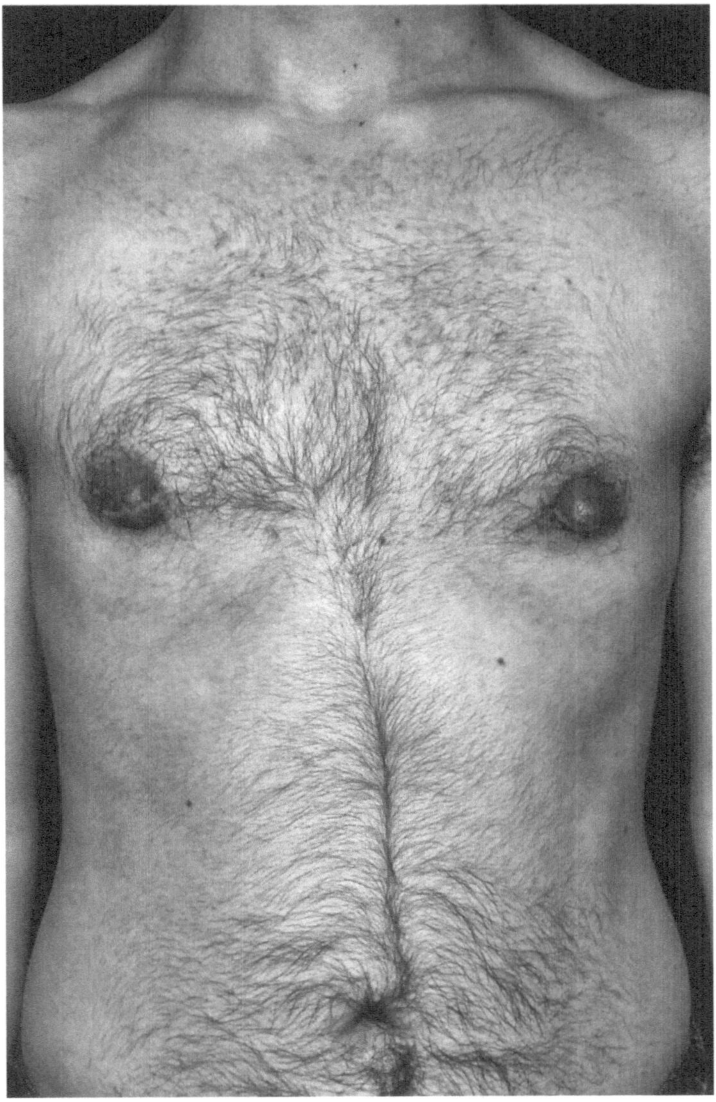

Figures 9.6a and 9.6b (continued)

incision is largely determined by the amount of breast ptosis, skin elasticity, and position of the nipple (Monstrey et al., 2008). Liposuction may be used as an adjunct to excisional techniques in order to remove excess fatty tissue. In general, the nipple-areola is re-positioned medial to the lateral border of the pectoralis major muscle. The postoperative management includes placement of closed-suction drains and external elastic compression.

Secondary revisions related to the scar and or nipple-areolar complex are not uncommon.

Masculinizing Genital Surgery

The goal of genital surgery in transgender men depends upon the goals of the individual. Surgery may range from clitoral release, metoidioplasty (surgical enlargement of the clitoris), with or without urethral lengthening in order to allow for voiding while standing, to a phalloplasty, capable of sexual penetration (Hage, van Turnhout, Dekker, & Karim, 2006).

Metoidioplasty, described in 1996 by Hage, is a less complicated alternative to phalloplasty (Hage, 1996). (See Figure 9.7.) The procedure entails

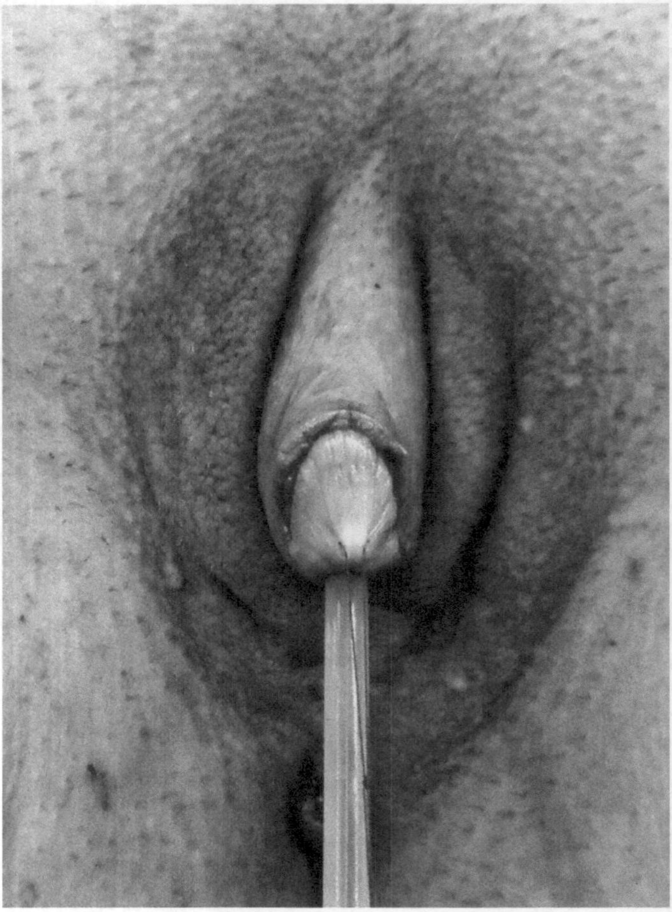

Figure 9.7 Metoidioplasty (photos used with permission of subject)

lengthening the hormonally hypertrophied clitoris by release of the ventral chordae and, when indicated, the suspensory ligament, and lengthening of the female urethra. Sexual penetration is generally not possible following metoidioplasty.

Most often, a hysterectomy and oophorectomy (removal of the ovaries) are performed at least two to three months prior to the metoidioplasty. The metoidioplasty procedure often involves concomitant removal of the female genitalia (vaginectomy) (Djordjevic et al., 2009). In the procedure, a portion of the vagina, incorporating the muscularis of the anterior vaginal wall may be used as a flap to reconstruct the fixed portion of the neourethra (Hage, Torenbeek, Bouman, & Bloem, 1993). The clitoral shaft is degloved and may be further released by detaching the suspensory ligament from the pubic bone. On the ventral aspect of the clitoris, the urethral plate is divided, allowing straightening and lengthening of the clitoris (Djordjevic et al., 2009). Additional lengthening of the urethra is performed with flaps developed from the labia minora.

Scrotoplasty, or creation of a neoscrotum, can be constructed with bilateral labia majora flaps at the time of metoidioplasty. Testicular implants are typically placed at a secondary surgical procedure to reduce the risk of infection and urethral complications. Individuals are hospitalized for several days for pain control and incisional care. Urination through the penis typically begins about three weeks after the procedure.

Complications following metoidioplasty include, but are not limited to, hematoma, delayed healing, infection, and urethral fistula and/or stricture.

Phalloplasty, or creation of a functional penis, represents the most complete genital transformation for transgender men. (See Figure 9.8.) Phalloplasty requires the use of either pedicled flaps (vascularized tissue) or free flaps. Pedicle flaps transfer tissue, typically from the thigh, groin, or lower abdomen to construct the penis, while free flaps involve the microsurgical transfer of tissue from a remote location. Similar to metoidioplasty, hysterectomy and oophorectomy are generally performed at least two to three months prior to phalloplasty.

The most common technique for penile reconstruction is the radial forearm free flap. This procedure transfers tissue, including blood vessels and nerves, from the forearm to reconstruct the penis and urethra. This flap allows single stage reconstruction of the urethra as well as a sensate phallus. Potential drawbacks of this technique include the visibility of the donor site on the forearm and the need for microsurgical skills. The anterolateral thigh flap is another technique for penile reconstruction. Similar to the forearm technique, tissue, including nerves, may be transferred from the thigh to construct the penis. Depending upon the individual's distribution of subcutaneous fat, a second flap may be required for urethral reconstruction. For both the forearm and thigh techniques, the urethra is formed by a skin-lined tube. As such, preoperative electrolysis may be required for depilation (hair removal) of the

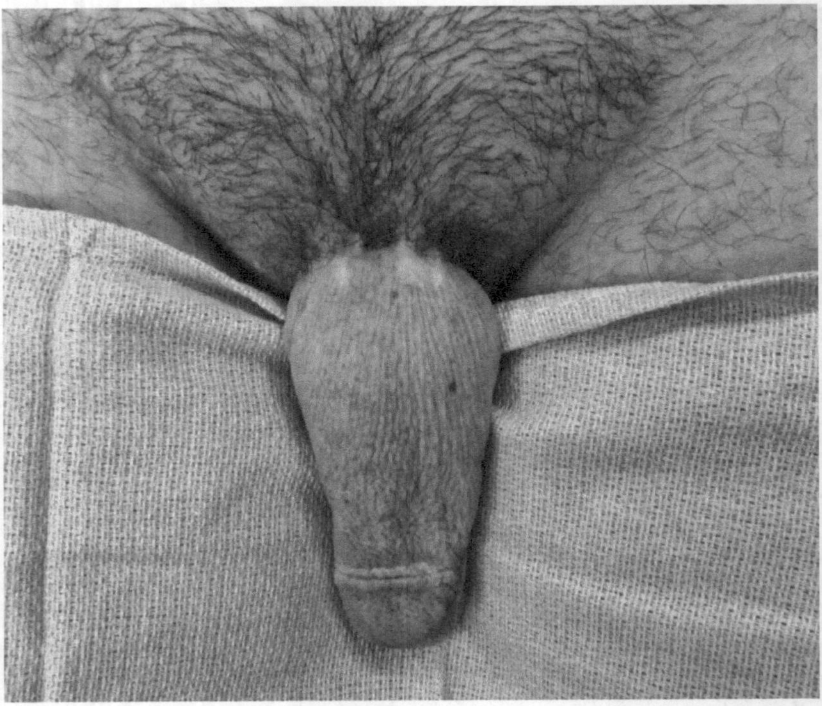

Figure 9.8 Phalloplasty (photos used with permission of subject)

elongated urethra. Additionally, skin grafting of the donor site (thigh or forearm) is required.

Additional phalloplasty techniques include the use of tissue from the back, known as the musculocutaneous latissimus dorsi flap. One notable downside of this flap is the lack of a sensory nerve to the tissue that will be used to construct the phallus. Additionally, the flap is often excessively bulky.

Following phalloplasty, individuals typically spend 7 to 10 days in the hospital for flap monitoring. Urination through the penis may begin several weeks after surgery, following either radiographic or cystoscopic assessment of the urinary tract.

Following phalloplasty, testicular implants and penile prostheses can be placed at a secondary procedure, allowing for penetrative intercourse. (See Figure 9.9.) While testicular implants may be placed several months following the phalloplasty, the penile prosthesis is typically placed 9 to 12 months after the initial procedure so as to allow the phallus to achieve protective sensation through reinnervation.

Complications following phalloplasty can be divided into early and late categories. Early complications tend be flap-related and include delayed wound healing and flap failure. Additional early complications include VTE,

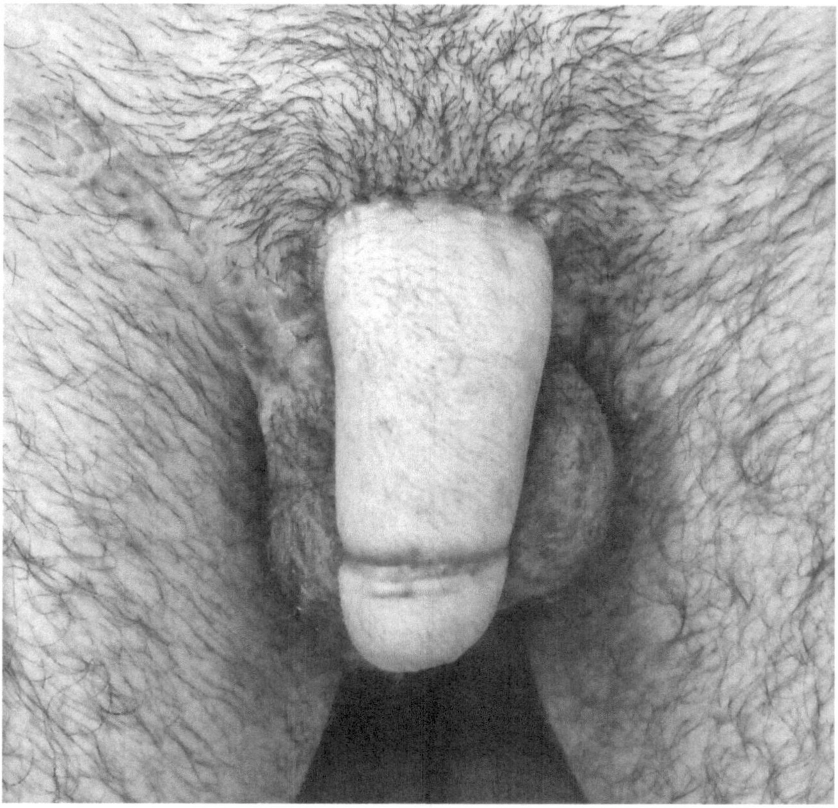

Figure 9.9 Phalloplasty with testicular implants (photos used with permission of subject)

bleeding, and infection. Most late complications are urologic in nature and include either stricture or fistulae. Additional complications are associated with testicular implants and penile prostheses. These complications may include infection, erosion, malposition, displacement, and mechanical failure.

Postsurgical Care

After genital surgery, individuals can resume hormone therapy once they are ambulating. Individuals are encouraged to wear dark, loose fitting clothing and avoid tight elastic straps at the groin region. Ambulation is encouraged and time spent sitting should be minimized so as to reduce perineal swelling. Patients are encouraged to elevate their legs as much as possible when sitting to aid with reduction of perineal edema.

It is recommended that individuals stay locally for several days after surgery if they live out of the area. Patients should travel with minimum baggage and, if possible, travel with a companion. Specific recommendations regarding travel (i.e., timing of air travel) should be discussed with the operating surgeon. For the first 6 weeks after surgery, activity is limited; patients should not lift more than 15 pounds or engage in strenuous exercise.

For ongoing mental health needs, individuals should continue treatment with their mental health professionals. Medical health care providers need to consider both the sex assigned at birth and transition gender when providing preventative care to transgender individuals. For example, transgender women may require screening for prostate disease as well as screening for breast cancer (Hembree et al., 2009). Transgender women who have undergone colonic vaginoplasty require speculum exam of the neovagina looking for evidence of gastrointestinal malignancy. For transgender men, evaluation of bone mineral density should be performed if risk factors for osteoporosis are present. In addition, if mastectomy/hysterectomy/oophorectomy are not completed, mammograms and annual Pap smear, as recommended by the American Cancer Society and American College of Obstetricians and Gynecologists, respectively, should be considered (Hembree et al., 2009).

Barriers to Gender Affirming Surgery

Although there is still work to be done, great strides have been made in removing barriers to care for transgender individuals. In 2014, The United States Department of Health and Human Services (HHS) repealed a 1989 decision declaring genital reconstruction surgeries for transsexualism "experimental." HHS ruled that "new evidence indicates that the ... rationale for considering the surgery experimental is not valid ... [and] new evidence indicates that transsexual surgery is a safe and effective treatment option for transsexualism in appropriate cases" (Department of Health and Human Services, 2014). Following this decision, Medicare beneficiaries became eligible for transgender care. In addition, an increasing number of third party payers have expanded coverage for gender affirming surgery when medically necessary. Some states now require insurance providers to cover some transition-related care. Coverage often follows the guidelines discussed in the *SOC*.

While coverage for genital surgery and masculinizing chest surgery are now covered with increasing frequency, breast augmentation, facial feminization, and tracheal shave are still often considered cosmetic procedures and not covered by insurance.

Individuals with private insurance who wish to proceed with surgery need written precertification from their insurance provider. Insurance plans typically follow the WPATH guidelines and request documentation, including referral letters from mental health providers, to verify that the requested surgery is medically necessary.

Case Examples

1. Jana is a 70-year-old transgender woman who has been living as a woman for 25 years. She has been taking spironolactone (androgen blocker) and estrogen for 20 years. Jana has worked with a psychologist and a social worker for several years to manage her gender dysphoria. She experiences depression and anxiety, both of which have been controlled for some time. Jana underwent facial feminization surgery and tracheal shave many years ago; the surgery helped improve her overall functioning. Jana and her mental health providers agree that vaginoplasty will help complete her transition and alleviate her gender dysphoria. In addition, her primary care physician confirms that she is medically fit for surgery. However, only recently has Jana been able to get coverage for surgery with her Medicare insurance. Jana is married and her partner is supportive of her desire to pursue vaginoplasty. During consultation, the surgeon reviews Jana's history, medications, and referral letters, examines Jana, and recommends penile inversion vaginoplasty. Jana's questions are addressed. Jana understands the risks involved in surgery and believes the benefits outweigh the risks. Jana is able to make an informed decision regarding vaginoplasty and would like to proceed. She understands that she will undergo hair removal, either by electrolysis or laser hair removal, in her genital area before surgery, and she will discontinue her hormone therapy two weeks prior to surgery. **Comment:** Psychiatric problems such as depression and anxiety are commonly seen in individuals with gender dysphoria. Provided these problems are under adequate control, they are not necessarily a contraindication to surgery. In addition, provided that individuals are in good health, age itself is also not a reason to withhold surgery. Research has suggested that adequate family and social support (in this case, a supportive partner) are important for postoperative functioning (Eldh, Berg, & Gustafsson, 1997).
2. Lee is a 17-year-old who prefers gender neutral pronouns such as "they" and "their." Lee has had persistent dis-identification with their sex assigned at birth. Lee has dysphoria regarding their breasts and has bound them for two years. Lee has consulted regularly with a therapist for more than one year. Lee's therapist, Lee's parents, and Lee all agree that pursuing chest or "top" surgery will help alleviate Lee's gender dysphoria. During consultation, the surgeon reviews Lee's history and referral letter, examines Lee, and makes recommendations regarding the technique for top surgery. Lee and Lee's parents understand the risks involved in surgery and believe the benefits outweigh the risks. They are able to make an informed decision regarding top surgery and would like to proceed. **Comment**: Some individuals younger than 18 years of age may be candidates for top surgery provided the individual, parents, and health care team concur that surgical care is appropriate.

3. Sam is a 45-year-old transgender man who underwent top surgery 6 years ago. He has been taking testosterone for 4 years. He now would like to proceed with genital surgery. Sam's main desire is to urinate while standing. He is not interested in penetrative intercourse at this time. Sam has followed regularly with a psychiatrist and a therapist. Sam and his mental health providers agree that genital surgery will help alleviate Sam's gender dysphoria. Sam has a BMI of 34 and has smoked half a pack of cigarettes daily for approximately 10 years. Besides these issues, Sam's primary care doctor believes he is medically fit for surgery. During consultation, the surgeon reviews Sam's history and referral letters, examines Sam, and discusses options for genital surgery. Given his desire to urinate while standing and his desire to avoid a procedure with donor site scarring, Sam would like to pursue metoidioplasty with urethral lengthening. The surgeon explains that phalloplasty will still be an option in the future should Sam's interests change. The surgeon counsels Sam to lose weight (BMI < 30) before surgery can be scheduled. In addition, Sam must quit smoking for at least 6 weeks prior to surgery. Urine continine will be measured prior to surgery, and the surgery will be postponed if the test demonstrates continued nicotine use. Some surgeons recommend holding testosterone for two weeks prior to surgery, although there is not consensus within the surgical community regarding this issue. **Comment**: Surgical options should be tailored to the needs of the individual. In this case, Sam's goal is to urinate while standing. Metoidioplasty with urethral lengthening, a less complicated procedure compared to phalloplasty, will be adequate. Importantly, Sam will still be eligible for phalloplasty in the future should he decide to pursue this option. Because obesity and smoking can negatively affect the surgical outcome, these issues need to be addressed prior to surgery.
4. Tyler is a 51-year-old transgender man who transitioned 20 years ago. He underwent chest surgery over a decade ago and has been taking testosterone since that time. He has desired to complete his transition with phalloplasty for years, but the cost was prohibitive. His insurance recently started covering the procedure and he is eager to proceed. Tyler's psychologist agrees that phalloplasty will be beneficial. Tyler has not seen a second mental health professional and reports there are no other gender specialists in his community. During consultation, the surgeon reviews Tyler's history and referral letter, examines Tyler, and discusses options for phalloplasty. Tyler's questions are addressed, and he would like to proceed with a radial forearm phalloplasty. Tyler understands that this is a staged procedure, and that he will require an additional surgery for placement of testicular implants and a penile prosthesis. Because Tyler needs a second mental health evaluation, the surgeon refers the patient for evaluation with a therapist who has expertise in gender care. **Comment:** The WPATH *SOC* serve as guidelines in providing care, but are not designed to be a barrier to care. In this case, Tyler appears to

be a candidate for phalloplasty, but he needs a second mental health evaluation. The surgeon facilitates a second evaluation with a gender specialist.

Conclusion

For many individuals with gender dysphoria, gender affirming surgery can be an important step in allowing them to become the person they know themselves to be. In order to optimize care, the surgeon must be a member of the interdisciplinary health care team, working closely with mental health and medical providers. With increased advocacy, awareness, and third party payer coverage, many transgender individuals are finally receiving the surgical treatment they need.

Take Home Points

- Some, but not all, transgender and gender non-conforming individuals desire surgery.
- Surgery options for transgender women include vaginoplasty, chest surgery, facial feminization, and tracheal shave.
- Surgery options for transgender men include chest surgery, metoidioplasty, and phalloplasty.
- Many insurance plans now cover gender affirming surgeries.

Recommended Reading

Hembree, W. C., Cohen-Kettenis, P., Delemarre-van de Waal, H. A., et al. (2009). Endocrine treatment of transsexual persons: An Endocrine Society clinical practice guideline.
Journal of Clinical Endocrinology and Metabolism, 94(9), 3132–3154.
Schechter, L.S. (2016). *Surgical management of the transgender patient.* New York, NY: Elsevier.
Schechter, L. S. (2016). Gender confirmation surgery: An update for the primary care provider. *Transgender Health, 1*(1), 32–40.

References

Department of Health and Human Services (2014, May 30). Departmental Appeals Board. Appellate Division. NCD140.3, Transsexual Surgery. Docket No. A-13-87. Decision No. 2576.
Djordjevic, M. L., Bizic, M., Stanojevic, D., Bumbasirevic, M., Kojovic, V., Majstorovic, M., . . . Perovic, S.V. (2009). Urethral lengthening in metoidioplasty (female-to-male sex reassignment surgery) by combined buccal mucosa graft and labia minora flap. *Urology, 74*(2), 349–353.
Eldh, J., Berg, A., & Gustafsson, M. (1997). Long-term follow up after sex reassignment surgery. *Scandanavian Journal of Plastic and Reconstructive Surgery and Hand Surgery, 31*(1), 39–45.

Ettner, R. (2007). *The etiology of transsexualism.* New York, NY: The Haworth Press.

Hage, J. J. (1996). Metaidoioplasty: An alternative phalloplasty technique in transsexuals. *Plastic and Reconstructive Surgery, 97*(1), 161–167.

Hage, J. J., Torenbeek, R., Bouman, F. G., & Bloem, J. J. (1993). The anatomic basis of the anterior vaginal flap used for neourethra construction in female-to-male transsexuals. *Plastic and Reconstructive Surgery, 92*(1), 102–108; discussion 109.

Hage, J. J., van Turnhout, A. A., Dekker, J. J., & Karim, R. B. (2006). Saving labium minus skin to treat possible urethral stenosis in female-to-male transsexuals. *Annals of Plastic Surgery, 56*(4), 456–459.

Hembree, W. C., Cohen-Kettenis, P., Delemarre-van de Waal, H. A., Gooren, L. J., Meyer, W. J., 3rd, Spack, N. P., . . . Montori, V.M. (2009). Endocrine treatment of transsexual persons: An Endocrine Society clinical practice guideline. *Journal of Clinical Endocrinology and Metabolism, 94*(9), 3132–3154.

Kanhai, R. C., Hage, J. J., Bloemena, E., van Diest, P. J., & Karim, R. B. (1999). Mammary fibroadenoma in a male-to-female transsexual. *Histopathology, 35*(2), 183–185.

Laub, D. (1999). Discussion: Augmentation mammaplasty in male-to-female transsexuals. *Plastic and Reconstructive Surgery, 104*(2), 550–551.

Lechien, J. R., Delvaux, V., Huet, K., Khalife, M., Piccaluga, M., Harmegnies, B., & Saussez, S. (2014). [Transgender voice and communication treatment: Review of the literature]. *Revue de Laryngologie - Otologie - Rhinologie (Bord), 135*(2), 97–103.

McIndoe, A. H., & Bannister, J. B. (1938). An operation for the cure of congenital absence of the vagina. *Journal of Obstetrics and Gynaecology of the British Commonwealth, 5*, 490–494.

McNeill, E. J. (2006). Management of the transgender voice. *Journal of Laryngology and Otology, 120*(7), 521–523.

Monstrey, S., Hoebeke, P., Dhont, M., De Cuypere, G., Rubens, R., Moerman, M., . . . Blondeel, P. (2001). Surgical therapy in transsexual patients: a multi-disciplinary approach. *Acta Chirurgica Belgica, 101*(5), 200–209.

Monstrey, S., Selvaggi, G., Ceulemans, P., Van Landuyt, K., Bowman, C., Blondeel, P., . . . De Cuypere, G. (2008). Chest-wall contouring surgery in female-to-male transsexuals: a new algorithm. *Plastic and Reconstructive Surgery, 121*(3), 849–859.

Schechter, L. S. (2009). The surgeon's relationship with the physician prescribing hormones and the mental health professional: Review for version 7 of the World Professional Association for Transgender Health's Standards of care. *International Journal of Transgenderism, 11*, 222–225.

World Professional Association for Transgender Health. (2011). *Standards of care for transsexual, transgender, and gender nonconforming people, Version* 7 (7th ed.). Retrieved from https://s3.amazonaws.com/amo_hub_content/Association140/files/Standards%20of%20Care%20V7%20-%202011%20WPATH%20(2)(1).pdf

10 Adjunctive Interventions

Supportive Services for Gender Role Transitions

Anne L. Boedecker, PhD

There is considerable controversy in the transgender community about the importance of "passing", i.e., being seen consistently as one's affirmed gender. At one time, it was the stated goal of nearly everyone who identified as transsexual (the applicable term at the time). A new generation of gender-variant individuals is challenging that assumption. For some, expressing themselves and being seen as gender non-conforming is preferable to moving from one "box" (binary identity) to the other.

Most transgender clients wish to change some aspects of their physical appearance. Their motivation, and the extent of their anatomical dysphoria, varies from individual to individual. Some transgender clients are looking to change their appearance to more closely match how they perceive themselves, and they care more about what they see in the mirror. Others want to live successfully "stealth" as their affirmed gender, and their focus may be on how others perceive them. There are others who do not attempt to alter their gender presentation out of lack of resources, or despair that they will ever pass. Other clients are happy with behavioral changes to their gender expression and will not seek medical interventions at all.

There are decisions that every transgender person needs to make about their physical transition: What is most important to me about my appearance? What do I want to see when I look in the mirror? What do I want others to see? How important is it for me to be attractive to potential partners? What degree of physical change is necessary for my career? What degree of physical change is my current spouse or partner able or willing to accept? What is realistic given my current age, body size, and shape? What funds do I have available for costly changes? What interventions are covered by my health insurance (if any)?

These issues are important to explore with your transgender clients. Those who change their appearance only for themselves may experience an alienating disconnection between their self-perception and how others see them. They may also experience unanticipated consequences. Given the current increase in gender policing in some parts of the country, gender non-conforming individuals, especially transwomen, are subject to increased discrimination, harassment and victimization (James, Herman, Rankin,

Keisling, Mottet, & Anafi, 2016). It may be helpful to guide your client through a risk/benefit analysis for their transition that includes these safety concerns.

Transgender clients who focus on how others perceive them face different challenges. They may become self-conscious to the point of hypervigilance. Some avoid going out in public dressed as their affirmed gender until they feel 100% sure of passing. Others continually seek an unrealistic standard of femininity or masculinity, subjecting themselves to multiple surgeries and/or dangerous hormone levels. They may need to be reminded that you do not have to be a beautiful woman or totally buff man to pass most of the time.

In any case, hormones and surgery alone will not always create the transformation that most clients need in order to reduce their gender dysphoria. There will always be some who are already feminine- or masculine-looking and acting and need little change in their appearance. If they start transitioning while young enough to take advantage of puberty blockers before masculinizing or feminizing hormone treatment, there will be little in the way of secondary sex characteristics to reverse. They may not need adjunctive interventions at all. Most transgender clients are not so fortunate. After the development of secondary sex characteristics, and the binary socialization as a man or woman, there is usually much work to be done in order to change a gender presentation that does not fit. Transgender clients who choose to transition late in life will have a lifetime of living in the role of their assigned gender and will have additional burdens in this regard.

To assist clients in developing their true sense of self in the world, mental health professionals need to be knowledgeable about the subtleties of gender presentation, without falling into the trap of stereotyping behavior. Providers also need to be informed about the adjunctive services that clients may need and be able to provide appropriate referrals. In urban areas, this may be relatively easy to do; in rural areas, it presents more of a challenge. After an explanation of gender presentation, and the services needed to refine it, ways to find them will be discussed. Dominant American cultural norms will be assumed, for the sake of general discussion, but these areas of intervention will also be applicable to other countries. Challenges of gender presentation vary in different cultures and sub-cultures, and those differences need to be taken into consideration. Therapists should, as always, be sensitive to racial, ethnic and sub-cultural norms in this area.

Gender Presentation and Attribution

Gender presentation is one aspect of social communication. We use other aspects of social communication when we flirt, for example, or behave during a job interview. Gender presentation is expressed in the way we dress, style our hair, walk, talk, and interact with others. It is both conscious—things we manipulate on purpose, like clothing and hair style, and unconscious—the way we move through a room, or subtle speech patterns. We are taught from an early age how to present ourselves in a way that conforms to our assigned gender. That training intensifies in adolescence and continues throughout adulthood. For example, there are dozens of magazines and TV shows devoted to showing us how to present ourselves successfully as a man or woman, and in these formats non-binary presentations are discouraged.

Gender attribution is how other people perceive us. In everyday life, we automatically "gender" the people we see (and hear) into binary categories. It is an automatic, unconscious process that happens in a split second. We do this based on a number of cues, such as voice, body shape, hair style, clothing, etc. Some cues are weighted more than others—the presence of large breasts is read as female and significant facial hair as male, generally overriding other ambiguous cues. Recognition of male and female faces is a subtle process that includes facial structure, coloring and contextual cues. In the absence of obvious cues, it is the overall impression that registers. It is the "preponderance of evidence" that matters. We are cognitively predisposed to resolve conflicting information and overlook what does not fit the general impression. Once we make that identification as male or female, it's set, unless there is a glaring inconsistency. For those with a non-binary gender identification this can make presenting one's true self even more complicated.

There are individual differences in what people pay attention to in gender-typing others. While it is impossible to predict how each person perceives gender, we can hazard a few generalizations. American teenage girls are more likely to notice the brand and style of jeans someone is wearing, while heterosexual men are predisposed to focus on body shape. That is one reason why a person in transition can walk through a shopping mall and be seen by some people as a man and others as a woman. The other people in the mall are noticing different cues and putting what they see into their own cognitive schema.

For those with binary identifications, it can take a lot of trial and error to learn how to present convincingly as a man or woman. This can be more challenging for transgender women due to stricter social constraints. Transgender men may have lived in "tomboy" mode for many years. It is important to remind clients who are transitioning that body image—how we perceive ourselves—changes more slowly than how others perceive us. This is because of the nature of perception. We do not always see exactly what is in front of us. We see what our brain perceives is there, which is based on a perceptual schema, a cognitive framework based on experience. Our brain automatically reverts to seeing ourselves in a familiar way. This is why people with anorexia can still see themselves as fat. Clients often see themselves as their former gender presentation far longer than others do.

Helpful Services for a Successful Transition

Voice and communication training is an important aspect of gender presentation. A common but false assumption is that only transgender women need voice training, and all they need to learn is how to raise the pitch of their voice. One estimate is that only 7% of communication is verbal, with 93% being non-verbal. There are documented differences in how men and women use speech, language, and non-verbal communication (Darn, 2005). There is evidence that some of these differences are biologically based. Most of the differences in how men and women use verbal and non-verbal communication, however, can be attributed to socialization. Our communication style has been greatly influenced by the social expectations of the gender we were assigned, within our particular culture. These are generalizations, of course, and reflect binary standards of masculine and feminine behavior. These differences may be more or less apparent in different settings and situations and in different sub-cultures.

A review of the current literature (Reiman, 2006–2013; 2014) suggests that American men and women tend to differ in:

1. proximity and use of space, with men claiming more space as their own and intruding more on women's personal space;
2. posture, position, and orientation to others in a conversation, with men standing and sitting with their legs farther apart and at an angle rather than facing directly;
3. body movements and gestures, with men moving more stiffly and women more smoothly;
4. physical contact, with women hugging each other more and using more comforting touch and men more likely to initiate firm or rough contact;
5. facial expression, with women both more expressive and better at reading facial expressions; and
6. use of eye contact, with men making less eye contact, unless they are trying to establish dominance, and women averting their eyes during conflict.

Gender differences also emerge in speech patterns and conversational style, particularly:

1. content of speech, with men limiting conversations to common topics, such as sports, and discussing facts more than relationships and feelings; women share more personal information, including feelings, and talk about topics in more depth;
2. vocabulary and sentence structure, with men using more commands than requests and more slang, and women using more descriptive language and politer speech;
3. conversational behaviors, with men more likely to disagree and debate, interrupt others, and assert their point directly; women tend to listen more attentively, give more non-verbal encouragers (e.g., nodding, smiling) and ask more detailed questions; and

4. purpose or motivation, with men communicating to make a point and assert their dominance; and women seeking to understand and be understood and enhance connection and cooperation.

Those subtleties of communication style are learned and can be unlearned. If your client is open and you as a therapist are willing to do some coaching, this can be incorporated into therapy sessions. It can also be part of voice feminization or masculinization training. Acting coaches can be valuable resources for transgender clients. If none of these are available encourage clients to observe and practice behavior more aligned with their gender identity.

Voice training is helpful for transgender clients who wish to change their voice and speech patterns. Men and women differ in several vocal qualities, although there is an overlap in what is recognized as a male or female voice. (This is good news especially for those with a non-binary identification). During puberty, the growth of male facial bones creates a larger vocal chamber, vocal chords grow longer and thicker and change position in the neck, and the larynx itself increases in size. These permanent changes give a male's voice its deeper pitch, resonance and loudness. In addition, there are typically gender-based speech differences in:

1. articulation, with women speaking more clearly and distinctly,
2. pacing and phrasing, with men speaking in shorter bursts and women in longer, more flowing phrases, and
3. intonation, with women using a greater range of pitch and thus a more melodic voice.

Putting all these differences together you can see why voice feminization or masculinization is more complicated than one might think. That is why good voice training is so important, especially, but not exclusively, for transgender women. Testosterone will thicken the folds of vocal chords in transgender men, thus lowering their voice. It does not change the size of the larynx and does not guarantee a deep resonant male voice (for more information, see Chapter 6). Feminizing hormone therapy for women cannot undo the physical vocal changes of puberty. The only sure way to develop a feminine voice is through training, and practice, practice, practice. This makes it one of the hardest challenges of transitioning from male to female.

Voice training should ideally be done with a speech and language therapist who specializes in voice feminization/masculinization. There are several CDs and programs available online, but there is no substitute for professional help. Specialists have the equipment necessary to test a person's pitch, and can tailor exercises to the client's unique needs. Finding a qualified speech therapist or voice coach can be challenging. Some clinics have group programs, and universities with speech pathology degrees may have students available. Otherwise it is a process of contacting speech therapists in your area and asking if they have experience with voice training. Singing coaches at music schools may also be helpful. Transgender men starting testosterone may be distressed by the quality of their voice as it changes. They may want to use a voice coach as well, especially to maintain their singing voice. Losing a good singing voice is a common concern, but less likely with practice and good vocal hygiene.

Social skills training is a related area that may need attention, in addition to communication skills. There is a shift in social expectations that comes along with a gender transition. Advice on how to behave in a public restroom falls in this category, as well as how to walk, sit, eat, shake hands, and generally carry oneself in a new gendered role. In addition, many transgender clients suffer from significant social anxiety and have few friends other than those they interact with online. No matter how you feel about social graces, offer or find assistance in this area if you feel it would benefit your client.

Hair styling is another important aspect of gender presentation. Hair style and the presence or absence of facial hair is one of the most obvious gender markers and one of the first that children recognize. For this reason alone, clients who are beginning a physical transformation are often encouraged to start with their hair. For feminization, hair growth and beard removal take time and also allow clients to see something changing in those impatient months before they start hormones or before the hormones have taken effect.

Clients choosing a more masculine gender presentation have often already adopted a short masculine hair style. Finding a short hair style that is age appropriate can be a challenge. Getting out a shaver and doing a buzz cut probably will not do it. Going to a men's barber can be daunting, and traditional hair stylists may not understand what the client is looking for. Helping clients find a transgender-friendly hair stylist is important. One of the possible effects of testosterone that transgender men are not always prepared for is male-pattern baldness. Asking them about the older men in their family, especially their maternal grandfather, will give them a chance to consider the odds that they will lose their hair sooner rather than later.

The only effective way for transgender men to grow facial hair is with long-term testosterone treatment. Theatrical make-up is expensive and time-consuming, and substitutes like dotting mascara on your face do not yield realistic results. Shaving does not promote hair growth, and minoxidil (Rogaine) is not approved for facial hair. Testosterone treatment will stimulate the growth of facial hair but is not guaranteed to produce a full beard. Some transgender men never develop more than a moustache and/or goatee. It depends on age, coloring, and genetic background; some genetic males cannot grow a full beard. It takes years, not months, for facial hair to develop fully, and it does not always grow in evenly. Hudson's FTM Guide (http://ftmguide.org/) has suggestions for beard and mustache styles.

Transgender women also have challenges with their hair. Unless they were able to start their transition at an early age and obtain puberty blockers they will most likely need additional services (described below). If your client has male-pattern hair loss, they have a bigger challenge. There are no miracle drugs or treatments that will grow a full head of hair back. Propecia® (finasteride) can help slow down hair loss but is not effective once you have lost a certain amount of hair. Hair transplants are an option for those who have minor hair loss, but they are expensive and painful. They can fill in a receding hair line and bring it forward, helping to minimize a masculine forehead. Often more than one treatment is necessary, but if done by a good surgeon the results are permanent and natural-looking. The cost depends on how much scalp you need covered, but the estimates start at $5,000 and go up.

Another viable option is a wig or hair piece. A good wig will balance the shape of a person's face and minimize masculine features. For best results a permanent wig should be carefully chosen and fitted by a wig specialist. Specialists tend to be very understanding and sensitive to their clients' needs, since they often work with women who have lost their hair due to chemotherapy. Ideally, you will be able to find a specialist who also has experience working with transgender women. A decent human hair wig costs from $100 to $500, and they will need two.

For some transgender women, hair feminization can be as simple as growing their hair long and finding a good hair stylist. These clients might need help finding transgender-friendly stylists and advice on how to maintain healthy hair. There are so many options for feminizing hair (color, highlights, curl/texture treatments); encourage your clients to experiment until they find what works for them. A good hair style frames the face to create an oval feminine shape.

In addition to hair styling, transgender clients may wish to take advantage of other salon services, such as manicures and pedicures, facials, and help with learning how to apply make-up effectively. There is an art and a science to using cosmetics not only to enhance a person's facial features but also contour their features to more closely resemble a feminine face. Not many transgender women can afford facial feminization surgery. Good make-up properly applied can make a big difference in a woman's confidence in how she presents. Some transgender women avoid using make-up, unfortunately, because of lack of knowledge and skill and/or shyness about learning. Estheticians, cosmetologists, Mary Kay (or other cosmetic company) representatives and most department store cosmetic counter assistants enjoy helping transgender clients look their best.

Hair removal is an expensive aspect of feminization. With the onset of puberty, male hormones start to change body hair from the soft fuzz of childhood to thicker, coarser, and generally darker hair. The development of facial hair comes later, but is generally completed by age 20. There is no way to reverse this process. Reducing testosterone and adding estrogen will have some impact on body hair, especially on the arms, legs, chest, and back. Body hair will get lighter and softer again, and easier to remove with shaving, waxing, or depilatories.

Facial hair is not affected by feminizing hormone therapy and will need to be removed with electrolysis and/or laser treatments. A combination of these two is often desirable; laser or flash lamp treatments provide an initial clearing, followed by months of electrolysis for lasting hair removal. This process will vary with the individual's skin tone and hair color, and can be best determined by a qualified professional. These treatments are most effective with darker hair, making transitioning later in life (when hair has turned gray or white) even more challenging. Caution your clients to be wary of anyone who promises quick results with these treatments. Be sure to ask the hair removal provider if they have worked with transgender people previously.

Laser is an approved method of *permanent hair reduction*. It works by disrupting hairs in the active growth cycle. Lasers designed for hair removal emit specific wavelengths of light that are absorbed by dark hair pigment. Typically, they work best when there is a high contrast between the (darker) color of the hair and the (lighter) color of the skin. It does not destroy the hair follicle, which is why it is not considered permanent hair removal. Because it only disables hair in the active growth cycle it needs to be repeated at regular intervals. Hair grows in three stages; only a certain amount will be in the active stage at any one time. Flash lamp treatments, such as IPL (Intense Pulse Light) have become popular because they are less expensive than laser methods. It is not technically a laser treatment, but it works in a similar way. IPL was developed for other types of facial treatments and does not use a specific bandwidth of light. It can potentially cause more skin damage than other methods.

All laser and flash lamp treatments must be done by qualified practitioners; in some American states, it must be done by or supervised by a physician. Practitioners can be found in salons, spas, and dermatologist offices. A good practitioner will be honest about which method will work best for an individual's hair and skin. Costs of laser and IPL treatments vary, depending on how much dark hair there is, the type of treatment, and the size of the area to be treated. A typical treatment "package" consists of 6–8 sessions spaced 6–10 weeks apart, with more as needed.

Electrolysis is the tried-and-true, time-tested method of hair removal; it has been around since 1857. It is the only method with FDA approval for *permanent hair removal*. Electrolysis works, as its name suggests, by targeting each hair follicle with an electrical current. It does not depend on hair color or skin color, so it can be used by everyone. It is, however, very painstaking. Given that the average person has 500–1000 follicles per square inch, it takes a lot of time to "clear" an area of facial hair. And given that a hair follicle can only be destroyed during an active growth phase, clearing must be done repeatedly.

Electrolysis can only be done by a licensed practitioner. (Home methods are not effective.) It is important to help clients find a skilled practitioner experienced working with transgender clients. Often providers are only familiar with female hair removal and unfamiliar with beard removal. Poorly administered electrolysis can result in scarring, hair regrowth, and infections.

Wardrobe assistance is another area often needed by clients undertaking a gender role transition. No matter how much we may believe in freedom of expression in gender presentation, there are times when we need to assist our clients in making appropriate wardrobe selections. Obviously, there are individual differences in style and how much a person cares about their wardrobe. But one of the biggest fears that transgender women express is looking like "a man in a dress." If your transgender client wants to blend in and dress appropriately you may either need to do some coaching yourself or help them find a wardrobe consultant.

The clothing and accessories we wear are a significant means of social communication. They carry not only cues about gender; they carry messages about who we are and what we are looking for from our audience. They communicate our personality and values, our social class, and even at times our profession or religion. Clothing communicates all this through color and style. Color is a powerful communicator and has been shown to affect the wearer's and the viewer's emotional responses (Terwogt & Hoeksma, 2001). Style includes fabric (texture, weight, and finish) and shape (cut, fit, and length). Once we learn the language of color and style, we can better express the message we want to send. And it has to be learned! Men may seem to have an easier time, with a narrower range of options, but how they dress also communicates clear messages about what they are all about, including their sense of masculinity and possibly sexual orientation.

Transgender women often need help in developing a full wardrobe. Those who have been "cross-dressing" for some time might need help switching from fancy evening attire to everyday clothing choices. A wardrobe analysis looks at the frequency of various activities over a week or a month and the clothes someone currently owns, then fills in the blanks with the types of outfits needed. If there are financial constraints, you can suggest basic mix and match pieces for work and a variety of accessories to go with them. Worksheets for wardrobe analysis and planning are available in *The Transgender Workbook: Your Journey to Womanhood* by Anne L. Boedecker. "Regular women" (as opposed to models and actresses) make decisions about what to wear based on:

1. Context. This includes activity, location, and occasion. Lunch with a friend at a country club calls for a different outfit than running errands, a job interview, or a night on the town. Social events have different formal or informal dress codes, which takes most women years to learn. Overdressing for an occasion can bring unwanted scrutiny.
2. Season and weather. This depends on local climate, but in most parts of the United States women need summer, winter, and in-between season clothing choices.
3. Their body type. The best way to avoid looking like a man in a dress is to wear clothing that fits well and creates the illusion of the "ideal" hourglass figure. There are resources on-line for how to best dress different body shapes.

4. Age and relationship status. Protest ageism all you like, but dressing like a teenager over a certain age stands out like a sore thumb. This may be challenging for women who have waited a long time to wear the clothes they have envied since they were young. It is a normal developmental stage to explore clothing choices in adolescence, but on an adult body some of those choices can look out of place. The same goes for clothing that shows a lot of skin, which can send an inaccurate message to observers, potentially even putting the client at risk for violence. Do not be afraid to caution your clients if what they are wearing is not appropriate for public presentation.
5. Coloring. Knowing what color "season" or "family" works best with different skin, hair, and eye colors can make a big difference in appearance. This applies to make-up choices as well.
6. Personal style. Clothing, jewelry, and accessories come together to create a style that's unique to individual women but can also be classified. These styles can be labeled various ways, such as sporty, artsy, classic, chic, urban, "boho", etc. That's where creativity comes in!

In some places there are image, wardrobe, and color consultants who specialize in this area; some of them work primarily with transgender women and crossdressers, others with women in general, and some specialize in working with men, others work with all people. Transgender women in professional jobs, or those who would just like to look more polished, would be well-advised to use their services. They are far more cost-effective than random shopping. Some boutiques and upscale clothing stores also provide shopping assistance. In addition, transgender women can benefit from a good bra-fitting session at a department store or lingerie boutique, as well as tips on using hip and buttock padding. Research these resources in your area in order to point your clients in the right direction.

Because women have more freedom in clothing choices than men, transgender men may have been dressing in masculine styles long before transitioning. But they too may need help in wardrobe planning and learning how to dress for their body type. There are challenges for transgender men and non-binary identified people too who want to avoid looking like a lesbian or like someone in male drag. The biggest challenges for transgender men are:

1. Finding clothes that fit. Learning about how men's pants are sized and finding the right sizes can be problematic. There are on-line sources, and a good tailor is an important resource.
2. Fitting a pear-shaped body with tree trunk-shaped clothes. There are tricks to minimizing hips and using the right clothing styles to create a more masculine shape.
3. Binders and packers. To fit into men's clothes without their breasts showing, most transmen choose to wear a binder to conceal their

breasts. For medical grade binders, transgender men are encouraged to talk with their primary care provider for advice. Over-the-counter products like ace bandages are not designed for this purpose (there is too much stretch), and by the time that good visual effect is achieved, breathing can be restricted. There are different types and styles of binders available on-line and there might be a period of trial and error to find ones that work best for your client; they will need two good ones so they will have one to wear when the other is drying after washing. Some transgender men also choose to "pack" their pants with a homemade or purchased prosthetic to create an appropriate bulge in their pants.

4. Transgender men also sometimes use shoe inserts for additional height; these can be found through on-line retailers.

Adjunctive Mental Health Services

No one changes their gender expression in a vacuum; we are all embedded in families, groups, organizations, and communities. As mental health professionals, we would be remiss if we did not address the impact of our client's transition on their relationships and the impact those relationships have on their transition. Being an advocate for your client and educating others in their circle or community is part of the role of the gender specialist. If your client is married or partnered, meeting with them and their significant other may be necessary. It is "cleaner," ethically speaking, to refer the family or couple to another gender specialist, but that is not always possible.

Couples and/or family therapy is often crucial for helping the client's family adjust to the transition, as well as helping the client come out to their family and assist the family over time. Parents, partners, and other family members typically progress through many of the aspects of the grief process: shock, denial, anger, bargaining, blame, and guilt, even depression. Children typically adapt well, but adolescents are often disturbed and burdened by the changes occurring in the family.

Spouses or partners often feel like their world has been turned upside down. Their reactions range from "Get out now!" to "This could be fun!" Even if they have known about their partner's gender variance, once the transition becomes public knowledge their social world changes. They often struggle with what the transition means for their sexual orientation. Couples therapy can help them sort out what kind of relationship (if any) they will have going forward. The ongoing relationship benefits if the partner is kept informed and allowed to express his or her feelings about the timing of various aspects of the transition. Consider including a spouse or partner in a session periodically.

Group therapy or a therapist-led support group is a tremendous benefit for anyone considering or embarking on a gender role transition. Although this is changing as more people become visible in the community, transgender clients have often lived in isolation from one another. Bringing them together provides support and promotes community-building and sharing of resources. This writer led a structured support group for transfeminine clients that ran continuously from 2002 until 2012. It met biweekly for many years, and then monthly; attendance ranged from two people to more than a dozen. The format included a time for check-ins, a discussion on a specific topic, and periodically a guest presenter. Topics included coming out to family, friends, and employers, legal identity changes and documents, coping with family around the holidays, shopping resources, surgery options, social skills, make-up, and accessories, and more. Invited guests included Mary Kay representatives, a speech therapist, and supportive spouses. New birthdays were celebrated, Halloween costumes encouraged, and a hilarious holiday party held every January.

Peer support groups for clients and family members are a valuable resource. Transgender support groups on campuses or at health clinics or elsewhere provide socialization, shared resources, and friendship. PFLAG (Parents and Friends of Lesbians and Gays (https://www.pflag.org) and SOFFA (Significant Others, Family, Friends, and Allies; http://transwellness.org/resources/support-and-community-resources/soffa/) groups offer support to family members as well. The advantage to the therapist-led support group is that the therapist can work with difficult group dynamics and keep the group from getting off-track. The advantage to the peer-led groups is the increased empowerment and autonomy.

Psychopharmacology/psychotherapy for comorbid conditions is another adjunctive therapy that is often useful or necessary for clients in transition. The World Professional Association for Transgender Health (WPATH) *Standards of Care* (2011) refer to ensuring significant mental health concerns are well-controlled before recommending hormone therapy. Many transgender clients present with significant anxiety, depression, and/or posttraumatic stress disorder in addition to their gender dysphoria. Proper assessment and treatment of these concerns is an absolute necessity. Referral to a transgender-friendly psychiatrist, psychiatric nurse practitioner, or knowledgeable physician when necessary is part of the scope of the gender specialist's practice. As distress associated with gender identity decreases, referral to providers trained in evidence-based psychotherapy for the comorbid conditions may also be indicated.

Summary

As noted in the WPATH *Standards of Care* (2011), a mental health professional is often called on to be an advocate, coach, and educator for transgender clients and their significant others. Given the number of additional services needed for transitioning, they must also develop referral resources for their clients. In large metropolitan areas, this can be as simple as researching transgender resources online. Sites such as Laura's Playground (www.lauras-playground.com/) and Hudson's FTM Resource Guide (http://ftmguide.org/) provide the names of physicians, surgeons, and other professionals throughout the country. In rural areas locating services can be more challenging. This writer has developed several strategies for developing a compendium of resources:

1. Collecting and displaying business cards from transgender-friendly service providers. This can be done by asking clients to bring in cards from those who have been helpful to them, or by soliciting cards from providers who have a good reputation.
2. Cold calls to important providers, such as endocrinologists and other physicians. Even if you can only reach a nurse at the office they will know if Dr. X sees transgender patients.
3. Encouraging peer-to-peer interaction. Introduce transgender clients with similar interests or concerns (with prior permission of course), or pair a more experienced client with a newcomer. Create a list of "big sisters" and "big brothers" willing to share their experience.
4. Promoting and supporting the development of peer support groups and networks. The therapist-led support group mentioned above became obsolete when a state-wide peer network was formed.
5. Contacting existing peer support groups and organizations for recommendations, or referring clients to them.
6. Maintaining a referral list. This is the most challenging method, as it needs frequent updates and revisions.

Over time, mental health professionals who work with transgender clients will accumulate a substantial list of service providers who are more than happy to work with transgender clients. The rewards of being a coach, mentor, advocate, and educator will be apparent in the results as they watch clients blossom into their true selves.

Take Home Points

- Gender presentation is a complex phenomenon, based on multiple cues. Transgender clients have important choices to make about when and how to change their gender presentation to more closely match their internal gender identity.
- Services needed for transforming physical appearance and gender presentation include:
    - voice and communication training
    - hair styling and hair removal
    - wardrobe and make-up assistance
    - socialization and social skills training
- Adjunctive mental health services include:
    - couples and/or family therapy
    - group therapy or therapist-led support groups

- peer support groups
- psychopharmacology/psychotherapy for comorbid conditions

- Mental health professionals serve as coaches, advocates, educators, and at times a clearinghouse of referral sources.

Recommended Readings

Boedecker, A. L. (2011). *The transgender guidebook: Keys to a successful transition.* Lexington, KY: Anne L. Boedecker.

Boedecker, A. L. (2015). *The transgender workbook: Your journey to womanhood.* Lexington, KY: Anne L. Boedecker.

Lev, A. I. (2004). *Transgender emergence: Therapeutic guidelines for working with gender-variant people and their families.* Binghamton, NY: The Haworth Press.

Wood, J. T. (2015). *Gendered lives: Communication, gender, and culture, eleventh edition.* Stamford, CT: CENGAGE Learning.

References

Darn, S. (2005). Aspects of nonverbal communication. *The Internet TESL Journal, XI*(2). Retrieved from http://iteslj.org/Articles/Darn-Nonverbal/

James, S. E., Herman, J. L., Rankin, S., Keisling, M., Mottet, L., & Anafi, M. (2016). *The report of the 2015 U.S. Transgender Survey.* Washington, DC: National Center for Transgender Equality. Retrieved from www.transequality.org/sites/default/files/docs/USTS-Full-Report-FINAL.PDF

Reiman, T. (2006–2013). Gender differences in communication. In *Gender Differences-Body Language University.* Retrieved from www.bodylanguageuniversity.com/public/213.cfm

Reiman, T. (2014, December 9). Body language and gender differences in communication. Retrieved from www.tonyareiman.com/articles

Terwogt, M. & Hoeksma, J. (2001). Colors and emotions: Preferences and combinations. *Journal of General Psychology, 122*(1), 5–17.

World Professional Association for Transgender Health (2011). *Standards of care for transsexual, transgender, and gender nonconforming people, Version* 7 (7th ed.). Retrieved from https://s3.amazonaws.com/amo_hub_content/Association140/files/Standards%20of%20Care%20V7%20-%202011%20WPATH%20(2)(1).pdf

11 Identity and Support Letters

Colt Keo-Meier, PhD
Kelly Ducheny, PsyD
Michael L. Hendricks, PhD, ABPP

The creation of support letters for transgender individuals' identity documentation and safe passage is a critical component of transgender affirmative care and an important professional competency. At its best, the creation and production of such letters is a form of advocacy and intervention. When done well, letters from providers can support and acknowledge individuals' gender identity and gender expression in powerful ways. These letters minimize clients' exposure to harassment and discrimination, reduce the likelihood of poor health outcomes, and normalize transgender identities for sources (e.g., police, workplace) receiving the documentation. As such, providers writing support letters have a critical hand in creating ever-wider pathways for transgender clients to access the care and respect they deserve without harm. When support letters are done poorly or left undone, mismatched documentation creates significant delays in accessing care, worsens transgender peoples' health outcomes, increases client anxiety, depression, and hopelessness, and may even place transgender people at greater risk of mistreatment by law enforcement officials and others. An inaccurate or absent support letter communicates that a client's needs are not a priority for the provider or health system, increases client distrust, reduces engagement in care, and leaves transgender people feeling trapped, isolated, angry, and confused. It can also create hesitancy and suspicion in systems slated to receive the documentation, raising concern that the requested action is not carefully considered or appropriate for the client or that the provider is unqualified to complete a support letter.

The purposes of supportive documentation are multifold. Letters serve to minimize intrusion, discrimination, and mistreatment of transgender individuals, to assist a client in accessing identity documentation that aligns with gender identity and gender expression, and to create safe passage through spaces and systems (e.g., airport security, public bathrooms, police stops, court, work places) that may not be transgender affirmative or aware. The World Professional Association for Transgender Health (WPATH) maintains that "documents matching self-identity are essential to the ability of all people to find employment, to navigate everyday transactions, to obtain health care, and to travel safely [....] Barriers to legal recognition for transgender and transsexual individuals may harm physical and mental health" (WPATH, 2015). Given its critical purpose, documentation must be created with an exacting awareness of the rules and requirements in specific geographic areas, with the fewest delays, and with the least intrusion in transgender people's lives and privacy.

The creation of supportive letters can be a time consuming but crucial task. Most of the time spent generating supportive documentation is not billable, necessitating the most efficient process possible given the frequent need for multiple types of supportive documents by many transgender clients. To most effectively create supportive documentation, a provider can create templates for each type of letter described in this chapter that are adapted to the requirements in the health care professional's specific geographic region. Most electronic health records (EHR) allow providers to save letter templates that can be auto-populated with client information. Providers should carefully attend to auto-populated items, such as legal name and salutations or pronouns, which may be mismatched in the EHR. Fortunately, letter templates can be customized as necessary before being printed and saved in the chart. Future EHR workflows will need to be developed to auto-populate a person's legal name in some places and their chosen name and pronouns in others. As EHRs become more sophisticated in documenting gender identity, pronouns, and chosen name, this will become easier. Computer-generated letters should always be produced on formal stationary and physically signed, preferably in blue ink, to demonstrate the authenticity of the letter and to reduce the chance that a letter may be declined. Given the frequency with which letter requirements change, as well as the differences in requirements across geographic regions, it is necessary to identify and regularly check reliable source information that tracks documentation requirements. In addition, it is strongly recommended that health care professionals identify transgender cultural advisors or informants who can regularly review templates to assure that documentation is respectful, accurate, and incorporates the evolving knowledge base in transgender health and identity.

Documentation for transgender people with a non-binary identity can be more complex to create given the lack of familiarity in many public systems with non-binary gender identity and gender expression. It is important to balance the depth of explanation of a client's unique identity with the purpose of the letter and the safety of the person moving through the system. Documentation should not over simplify a client's identity but should offer the least information necessary to facilitate the purpose of the letter while helping the reader of the letter feel calm and supportive of the client. Several countries, including Australia, Bangladesh, Denmark, India, Nepal, and New Zealand now offer a legal documentation alternative sex option beyond male and female, such as X or Other. In the United States (U.S.), Oregon was the first state to offer a legal, non-binary sex identification option in 2016 for use on state-specific documents.

In general, a broad range of health care providers can submit supportive documentation, including but not limited to physicians, nurse practitioners, physician assistants, psychiatrists, endocrinologists, psychologists, social workers, and professional counselors. Some forms of documentation require specific credentials (e.g., U.S. passport letters require a physician's signature). In this chapter, we discuss three main types of non-surgical documentation that providers will likely encounter on a regular basis: federal or national documentation, which includes requests to alter the gender marker on a person's passport or social security card; state documentation, which includes requests to alter the gender marker on a person's birth certificate and driver's license, and for name change; and safe passage letters. Given the dramatic variety of documentation requirements across different countries, this chapter will primarily address requirements in the U.S. Providers in other countries can still make excellent use of the guidance and letter templates provided but are advised to review the legal requirements in their countries and consult with experienced letter writers to best guide their advocacy efforts on clients' behalf.

Federal or National Documentation

Federal or national support letters are typically short and specific. This documentation consists of a letter to change the gender marker on a client's national passport or social security card. Language on the passport letter should not be varied from the standard format given the strict requirements in place, since even small alterations can result in refusal and return of the documentation or the issuance of a limited-validity, 2-year passport rather than a full-validity, 10-year passport. U.S. regulations require that the letter must be signed or co-signed by a physician. At this time, U.S. regulations require that the "new gender" of the client be identified as male or female. Documentation will be returned unprocessed if an alternate gender is requested. As gender identity options that are recognized by the federal government evolve, this will change.

U.S. Passport/Social Security Administration Letter

[DATE]

To Whom It May Concern:

I, Marcus Smith, MD, am the attending physician for [CLIENT LEGAL NAME (DATE OF BIRTH)], with whom I have a physician/patient relationship and whom I have treated. [CLIENT LEGAL NAME] has had the appropriate clinical treatment for gender transition to the new gender, female.

I declare under penalty of perjury under the laws of the United States that the foregoing is true and correct.

Sincerely,

[SIGNATURE]

License Number: 123456789, Wisconsin

U.S. State Documentation

U.S. state documentation letters are typically longer than federal documentation letters. More importantly, requirements for content vary by state and sometimes even by county within the same state. The National Center for Transgender Equality has compiled an online ID Document Center (www.transequality.org/documents) with relevant information for each state's driver's license and birth certificate revision requirements. There is no uniform name change or gender marker change process for birth certificates or driver's licenses in the U.S.; each state or county has its own stipulated requirements. However, one constant across all U.S. states is that name changes always require a court order. Given the wide variety of requirements across different geographic regions and the distances some transgender clients travel for affirmative care, health care providers must often learn and apply the requirements of several jurisdictions in their support letters. In addition, geographic differences in documentation requirements and the way different forms of identification are then sequentially affected can dictate different recommended sequences for documentation revision (e.g., name change court order obtained first, so a driver's license will show the new name when a gender marker change is requested).

Navigating legal systems can be complex and may require legislative advocacy by providers and health systems to reduce barriers and outdated legislative requirements. For example, in Illinois, the American Civil Liberties Union (ACLU), Lambda Legal, medical/behavioral health providers and legal counsel at Howard Brown Health (an LGBT health center), and other advocates collaborated with state officials to revise proposed legislative language to facilitate gender marker change on Illinois birth certificates. Proposed language was drafted that, if accepted, would remove the requirement of surgical interventions and instead base the approval for an Illinois birth certificate gender marker change on documentation submitted by a medical or behavioral health care provider, consistent with WPATH (2015) recommendations. The proposed language also expands the types of providers who can offer such documentation to include medical and behavioral health providers who hold an independent license to practice, including physicians, nurse practitioners, physician assistants, psychiatrists, psychologists, social workers, marriage and family therapists, and professional counselors. If approved, transgender people in Illinois will have significantly fewer barriers and costs associated with a birth certificate gender marker change in the future. While such legislative initiatives can take years, transgender clients greatly benefit from strategic guidance and community ingenuity in meeting specific geographic requirements that are restrictive or difficult to navigate.

Some jurisdictions have revised the procedures for changing the gender marker on driver's licenses and similar state documents so that a letter is no longer needed or even accepted. In these U.S. states, the state agency that issues driver's licenses may have a form that must be filled out by the applicant which requires that a licensed health care professional simply check the appropriate box and sign. In most of these jurisdictions, forms are accessible online. An example is the form currently required by the Virginia Department of Motor Vehicles: www.dmv.state.va.us/webdoc/pdf/dl17.pdf. Other states, such as Illinois, only require a safe passage letter signed by a licensed health care professional to alter the gender marker on a driver's license. It is important to note that changing the name on a state identity document typically requires submission of a court order or copy of a federal identity document (e.g., passport) and that most states require that the name be changed on all documents within 30 or 90 days of obtaining the name change court order.

In U.S. jurisdictions in which a letter is still required to change the gender marker on a state identity document, requirements can vary. In Texas, the transgender community has encountered several barriers to name and gender marker changes. In this state, both name and gender marker changes require a court order and may be handled in different courts (e.g., family court or civil court). Some judges automatically deny requests for both name and gender marker changes by transgender people, while others will only grant name changes. Once one judge has denied a person's petition, it becomes much more challenging to find another judge to overturn the previous determination.

To address these barriers, the Texas transgender community has banded together to find willing judges. Community members and advocates have found that filing in counties with judges known to approve requested changes is most effective and will advise other transgender people to travel out of their county if necessary to access the needed court orders. If a transgender person is concerned that another citizen will object to their name or gender marker change, the transgender person may be advised to wait a certain number of days (e.g., 30) before sharing news of the change until the court order is finalized. Once it is finalized, the name change cannot be protested.

Sample Name and Gender Marker Change Letter

[DATE]

Re: Aydin Michael Jones

Legal Name: Ashley Michelle Jones

To Whom It May Concern:

I am a licensed psychologist who has expertise in working with issues of gender identity and expression. I am a member of the interdisciplinary transgender health team at the Forest Center for Health and of the ABCD Professional Association. **The purpose of this letter is to support Aydin Jones's request to have the gender on his legal documentation changed from FEMALE to MALE and to have his name changed from Ashley Michelle Jones to Aydin Michael Jones.**

It is my professional opinion, based upon my psychological assessment of Aydin, that he should be legally recognized by his chosen name of Aydin on all identification documents. This change is a critical and positive part of Aydin's gender transition and is expected to result in improved health and well-being. My professional opinion is informed by the World Professional Association for Transgender Health (WPATH) *Standards of Care*, 7th Edition (WPATH, 2011). A delay in Aydin's documentation changes may have a serious negative impact on Aydin's personal safety and treatment in public places, and may harm his physical and mental health (WPATH, 2015). Legally recognized identification documents that match a person's self-identity are necessary for all people to find employment, to navigate everyday transactions, to obtain health care, and to travel safely; a person's transgender status should not preclude them from enjoying the legal recognition all citizens expect and deserve (WPATH, 2015).

In my professional opinion, it would be harmful to Aydin's well-being to have his legal name and gender change on his documentation denied.

By signing this letter, I swear or affirm under penalty of perjury that the information is true and correct.

[SIGNATURE]
Chris S. Houston, Ph.D.
Forest Center for Health
Springfield, Ohio
513-555-1212

Safe Passage

Among the identity and support letters clinicians are likely to write, safe passage letters are the most personalized and most complex. Each letter must be tailored not only to the specific individual for whom it is written, but also to the circumstances for which that individual anticipates needing a letter. The range of circumstances is broad and encompasses travel, interaction with law enforcement, gym or locker room use, educational pursuits, and employment. The purpose of a safe passage letter is to provide a document that can be presented to authorities (e.g., police, airport security, customs, gym staff, employers, school officials) when there is a need for clarification of a person's gender or gender presentation or when there is a need for guidance on appropriate treatment of that person. The goal of the letter is to provide the person in authority with information that facilitates respectful treatment in a variety of situations. To accomplish this, the health care professional must write a letter that can be understood by people who may be unfamiliar with gender identity, transgender people, and issues faced by transgender people when moving through different systems. The letter must be non-threatening and offer respectful instruction to the person in authority.

While two safe passage letters are offered below, these letter templates will not be universally applicable and will need to be adapted to each person's unique needs. Because safe passage letters will not necessarily be used in just one jurisdiction, the language used in these letters should anticipate the most restrictive rules and procedures in the surrounding jurisdictions. Depending on the jurisdiction, a safe passage letter may need to include language that an individual *must* demonstrate their specific gender expression *in all situations*.

This language may better satisfy especially restrictive requirements and offer a compelling rationale for the transgender person's appearance and requested actions (e.g., bathroom and pronoun use). Similarly, some safe passage letters may include a statement articulating the person's requirement to demonstrate their gender expression given that some jurisdictions still require a specified period of lived experience to approve a gender marker or name change, even though the WPATH *Standards of Care* (2011) no longer requires specific time-frames.

Safe Passage Letter (Binary Gender Travel)

[DATE]
Re: Sarah Nguyen
Legal Name: Sean Nguyen
To Whom It May Concern:

This letter serves to advise you that the above named individual is a transgender client in my clinical care. Sarah Nguyen, also known as Sean Nguyen, is under my care and is undergoing a medically supervised treatment to transition from the assigned sex of male to female. She presents as female, as is appropriate to her gender identity, and living as a woman in all environments is a required component of her treatment.

During transition, Sarah may present with a mixture of male and female characteristics (breast development, face shape, body or facial hair, tone of voice, etc.) which may leave some people confused about her gender. This is normal and must be allowed as Sarah makes her gender transition. Sarah is unable to legally change the gender designation on her personal identification until completion of the transition process. Until that time, her legal identification may not match her appearance. This is not in Sarah's control and represents no intention to misrepresent herself. She should be treated with utmost respect and protection from discrimination and harassment.

Sarah identifies as a transgender woman and should be afforded the same basic human rights as other women, including being referred to with the pronouns of she, her, and hers, and using the women's bathroom and locker room facilities. While Sarah may identify as transgender, this has no implications for her mental stability or competence. Sarah is a high functioning and emotionally stable individual.

To authenticate that this letter is indeed for the person before you, a description of Sarah is included. She is approximately 74 inches/188 cm tall, has short brown hair and brown eyes. Her birthdate is August 12, 3456 and driver's license number is 12345678.

If there are any questions or concerns related to the authenticity of this letter, please feel free to contact me directly at 415-555-1212. Please be advised that I can provide general information about letters like this and my experience, but I will not be able to discuss any specific information with you about Sarah without her written permission. Any assistance you can offer her in her travels would be much appreciated. Thank you in advance for your professional and respectful treatment of Sarah.

By signing this letter, I swear or affirm under penalty of perjury that the information is true and correct.
Sincerely,
[SIGNATURE]
Sean Whitlock, Psy.D.
San Francisco, California
415-555-1212

A further challenge in writing safe passage letters occurs when writing on behalf of an individual whose gender identity or expression falls outside of the gender binary. Professional guidelines acknowledge that gender is not inherently binary (e.g., American Psychological Association, 2015), but this fact challenges the societally enforced conceptions of gender as consisting of only male and female and being automatically aligned with sex assigned at birth. Even in today's social climate of increased awareness of transgender people, letters for those who present with or who have a non-binary identity necessitate a more detailed explanation of that person's experience. While health care professionals are strongly encouraged to work collaboratively with their clients in writing the narrative of a safe passage letter, with non-binary clients, collaboration is essential. In doing so, it is of utmost importance to address situations in the letter that the individual expects to encounter. For these reasons, actual letters will vary widely, depending on the individual and the purpose of the letter.

Safe Passage Letter (Non-Binary Gender, Bathroom Use, and Identification Document Discrepancies)

[DATE]
Re: Brynn Thompson
Legal Name: Brian Thompson
To Whom It May Concern:

This letter serves to advise you that the above named individual is a transgender client in my clinical care. Mx. Brynn Thompson, also known as Brian Thompson, is under my care and is undergoing a medically supervised gender transition treatment. Mx. (pronounced "mix") is the gender-neutral version of Mr. or Ms. When addressing or referring to Brynn please use the pronouns they/them/theirs.

I have thoroughly evaluated Brynn and have determined that their gender is not male or female, but is instead a mixture of genders and presentations. Brynn is receiving medically necessary care in accordance with internationally recognized standards to transition from the assigned/biological sex of male to a different gender identity.

When someone is making a gender transition, they often present with a mixture of female and male characteristics (breast development, face shape, tone of voice, body or facial hair, etc.), which may leave some people confused about this person's gender. This is normal and must be allowed as Brynn makes their gender transition. Brynn should be treated with utmost respect and protection against harassment and discrimination.

Brynn identifies as a non-binary transgender individual and should be afforded the same basic human rights as other people, including being referred to with the pronouns of they/them/theirs, and using the bathroom or locker room facility that is safest for them. In some cases, the female facilities will be the most appropriate and, in other cases, the male facilities will be safer. Brynn is able to make the best decision each time they choose which gender-segregated space they enter and should not be harassed or asked to leave either space. While Brynn may identify as transgender, this has no implications for their mental stability or competence. Brynn is a high functioning and emotionally stable individual.

This letter serves as an official document for Brynn to explain the discrepancies between their name, appearance, or gender marker (M or F) on their identification or other official documents. Aspects of their legal identification may appear discrepant. This is not in Brynn's control and represents no intention to misrepresent themselves.

To authenticate that this letter is indeed for the person before you, a description of Brynn is included. They are approximately 74 inches/188 cm tall, have long wavy hair, and green eyes. Their birthdate is August 12, 3456 and driver's license number is 12345678.

For your understanding of my qualifications to write this letter, I am a licensed psychologist at General Hospital who has expertise in working with issues of gender identity and expression. I am a member of the ABCD Professional Association and am aware of the laws that protect transgender people and the basic rights to which they are entitled. The majority of clients I serve are transgender.

If you have any questions regarding the statements I have made or the authenticity of this letter, feel free to contact me at 410-555-1212. Please be advised that I can provide general information about letters like this and my experience, but I will not be able to discuss any specific information with you about Brynn without their written permission. Thank you in advance for the professional treatment and care you will provide to Brynn.

By signing this letter, I swear or affirm under penalty of perjury that the information is true and correct.

Sincerely,
[SIGNATURE]
Miguel Maldonado, Psy.D.
General Hospital
Providence, Rhode Island
401-555-1212

Take Home Points

- Support letters for transgender individuals' identity documentation (state and federal or national) and safe passage are critical components of transgender affirmative care.
- Well-written letters can be profoundly assistive and affirming; poorly written or uninformed letters can do harm.
- Letters for U.S. federal or national documentation changes are short, specific, and must be signed by a physician.

- State documentation letter requirements are much more complex. Each U.S. state, for example, and sometimes each county, has different requirements for changes in name and gender.
    - All name changes throughout the U.S. require a court order.
    - Some U.S. states require a court order for gender marker changes, while others do not.
- Safe passage letters are the most personalized and complex. These letters serve to create safe passage through spaces and systems (e.g., airport security, public bathrooms, police stops, court, work places) that may not be transgender affirmative or aware.
- Letters for people with non-binary identities are more complex and nuanced to write.
- Providers are encouraged to collaborate with transgender clients to create accurate and affirming letters that create pathways for them to access the care and respect they deserve without harm.
- Advocacy efforts by mental health professionals to revise outdated, overly restrictive or non-affirming requirements to access name and gender marker changes can be effective in removing or reducing barriers transgender people experience.

Recommended Reading

Singh, A. A., & dickey, l. m. (Eds.) (2017). *Affirmative counseling and psychological practice with transgender and gender nonconforming clients*. Washington, DC: American Psychological Association.

References

American Psychological Association (2015). Guidelines for psychological practice with transgender and gender nonconforming people. *American Psychologist, 70*(9), 832–864.

World Professional Association for Transgender Health. (2011). *Standards of care for transsexual, transgender, and gender nonconforming people, Version* 7 (7th ed.). Retrieved from https://s3.amazonaws.com/amo_hub_content/Association140/files/Standards%20of%20Care%20V7%20-%202011%20WPATH%20(2)(1).pdf

World Professional Association for Transgender Health. (2015). *WPATH statement on identity recognition*. Retrieved from https://amo_hub_content.s3.amazonaws.com/Association140/files/WPATH%20Statement%20on%20Legal%20Recognition%20of%20Gender%20Identity%201-19-15.pdf

12 Finding Additional Resources

Zander Keig, LCSW, MSW, MS
Jamison Green, PhD, MFA

The views expressed herein are those of the authors and do not necessarily reflect the official policy or position of the Department of the Navy, Department of Defense, or the U.S. Government.

Mental health professionals who work with transgender clients are strongly encouraged by the World Professional Association for Transgender Health (WPATH) *Standards of Care* (SOC) (2011) to develop professional peer networks within which they can discuss complex cases, share information about the field, and increase their exposure to the variety and patterns of experience and expression they may observe throughout the transgender community. Clients frequently will ask mental health professionals for referrals to community-based resources, legal advisors, governmental services, other health care providers (e.g., endocrinologists, surgeons, speech therapists for vocal coaching), and many other information resources. Even for health care groups where such services are currently available within the organization, the availability of care is often dependent on one or two trained individuals—who might become unavailable at any time—so, developing a community of practice that includes external resources is important.

Any published list of resources may quickly become outdated. Therefore, we present here a general approach to finding clinical resources and appropriate training materials for the individual mental health professional and for the treatment team. We also offer recommendations for identifying community-based resources and other supports for clients.

Finding Mental Health Colleagues

Joining professional associations where lesbian, gay, bisexual, and transgender (LGBT) or transgender-specific care is a primary focus is probably the best way to make connections with experts in the field of transgender health. Members of these groups very likely can refer you to colleagues in your own geographic area or inform you about newly published research and upcoming conferences on transgender health topics. They can also tell you what journals, online resources, or listservs they regularly monitor. Many professional organizations offer special interest subgroups for LGBT or specifically for transgender issues, and joining subgroups within your current professional memberships is a great place to start.

The World Professional Association for Transgender Health (WPATH) was incorporated in 1979 and was originally named the Harry Benjamin International Gender Dysphoria Association (HBIGDA) in honor of Harry Benjamin, MD (1885–1986), one of the first physicians to work with transgender clients. WPATH is a global, interdisciplinary, professional membership organization that hosts a biennial international scientific symposium and offers regional chapters which host their own biennial conferences in the alternate years. Check the WPATH web site (www.wpath.org/) for more information and for links to regional group events. By discipline, the highest percentage of WPATH members are mental health providers (WPATH, 2016).

WPATH provides the premier networking private email lists in the field of transgender health—both regional and international—where members can ask any question and can be assured that they will be answered in a helpful way. This member benefit, along with discounts on conference registration, continuing education credits, and the opportunity to earn WPATH professional certification, is probably one of the most widely appreciated. Members may also access an online directory, where they can search for members by name, location or specialty, among other search options. Virtually all leading practitioners in the field of transgender medicine and mental health are members of WPATH.

With more on the way, WPATH's sister regional professional associations and regional affiliate groups currently include:

- Australia/New Zealand Professional Association for Transgender Health (ANZPATH)
- Canadian Professional Association for Transgender Health (CPATH)
- European Professional Association for Transgender Health (EPATH)
- US Professional Association for Transgender Health (USPATH)

In addition to WPATH, the institutions and organizations listed below provide continuing education, host annual conferences on transgender health and provide further opportunities to network with other professionals.

- The University of California, San Francisco (UCSF) Center of Excellence for Transgender Health offers capacity-building programs, community-based research resources, program evaluation and technical assistance, and provides cutting-edge primary care information through its Primary Care Protocols Project (online at www.transhealth.ucsf.edu/). In addition, the Center of Excellence for Transgender Health hosts the National Transgender Health Summit (http://transhealth.ucsf.edu/summit) in Oakland, CA, alternating years with the WPATH scientific symposium.

- The annual Philadelphia Trans Health Conference offers a Trans Behavioral Health Initiative Track (https://www.mazzonicenter.org/trans-health) that provides a broad selection of workshops and panel discussions to increase awareness of transgender, transsexual, and gender non-conforming individuals' experience.
- Gender Diversity Education and Support Services, which hosts the Gender Odyssey Professional Conference (www.genderdiversity.org/gopro), provides two opportunities (Los Angeles, CA and Seattle, WA) for clinicians to acquire knowledge pertaining to working with transgender clients from all age groups (children to seniors).
- Association for Lesbian, Gay, Bisexual, and Transgender Issues in Counseling—ALGBTIC (www.algbtic.org/), a division of the American Counseling Association, offers members access to a listserv, holds an annual conference, maintains a Transgender Committee (www.algbtic.org/transgender.html) and also makes available a useful article, "Competencies for Counseling Transgender Clients," which may be downloaded from the Competencies page on their web site.
- Swiss Transtagung—Trans Swiss Conference (https://transtagung.tgns.ch/) is a two-day conference in Bern covering a wide array of transgender topics: documentation changes, youth, post-transition, surgery abroad, parents and partners, genderqueer, disclosure, handling the media, hormones, and much more.
- This Trans Conference Guide (http://transguys.com/?s=conferences) provides an extensive, though not exhaustive, list of conferences in the United States, Canada, and Europe.

This list may be updated in future years, but even in its limited form it may be a starting point for Internet searches to locate recurring or new conferences.

Connecting with Other Disciplines (Building a Local Team or Network of Providers)

Because WPATH is interdisciplinary, mental health professionals surely will encounter providers from other disciplines in the field of transgender health, but when your clients need referrals, it can be difficult to find them in one's own backyard. Transgender issues are increasingly the subject of various academic and professional conferences, and transgender-focused specialties are developing as academic topics within Gender Studies or Transgender Studies departments at colleges and universities. The topic is also gaining attention within other medical specialty conferences such as those focused on urology, gynecology, nursing, primary care, and plastic surgery. Continuing education programs are increasingly available in the areas of transgender families (generally for parents with transgender children), law and policy-making, and spirituality. Below are some examples of conferences where cross-discipline networking is offered and encouraged.

- Trans* Studies: An International Transdisciplinary Conference on Gender, Embodiment, and Sexuality (https://www.lgbt.arizona.edu/transgender-studies-initiative-main) held in Arizona is "Working with professors, researchers, and students across disciplines and borders, [to] develop resources, programming, and exchanges of information."
- The Centre for Gender Studies/Centrum för genusforskning (GCF) in Sweden (https://www.kau.se/en/centre-gender-studies/research/transgender-studies) "is one of the first European institutions which include Transgender Studies as one of its main areas in respect to research and teaching that regularly stages international workshops, research residencies, conferences and seminars, organised on a regular basis by researchers as well as students."
- Moving Trans* History Forward (www.uvic.ca/mthf2016/) is a Canadian conference where "Trans and gender non-conforming (GNC) community-based scholars and activists, academics, archivists, librarians, family members, and allies of trans and GNC people explore preserving and recounting the history of trans and GNC people and communities in all eras and regions of the world."
- Gender Studies Network called GEXcel (the International Collegium of Transdisciplinary Gender Studies, www.gexcel.org/), is "a collaboration between 3 Swedish universities, working together with world leading scholars in the diverse field of Gender and Feminist Studies."
- Transgender Lives: The Intersection of Health and Law Conference (www.transadvocacy.org/transgender-lives-conference)—This conference, based in Connecticut "seeks to raise awareness of the interconnectivity and interdependence of two critical areas to the lives of the trans and gender non-conforming individuals."
- Gender Spectrum (https://www.genderspectrum.org/), located in Emeryville, CA, provides a wealth of sophisticated material designed to support parents and clinicians in understanding and supporting their transgender children, teens, and clients (whether they are the children or the parents). The organization also hosts an annual conference for parents and clinicians, and their staff can be contracted with to deliver educational presentations about gender to schools and other audiences around the United States (U.S.), and possibly beyond.

Community-based social events will sometimes include an educational or health care aspect. A Google search of "Transgender Community Events" yielded over 28,000 results. Here are some examples from this search:

- Houston (U.S.) Transgender Unity Banquet (www.unitybanquet.com/)—"Presented by the Houston Transgender Unity Committee (HTUC) and has become the largest Transgender Community event held in Houston, Texas each year. The Banquet raises money for scholarships,

Houston Pride activities, Houston Transgender Day of Remembrance (TDOR), annual recognition awards, and small grants."

- International Transgender Day of Remembrance (https://tdor.info)—This annual event, held in cities across the U.S., Canada, Europe, and Australia, on or around November 20 occurs "to memorialize those who were killed due to anti-transgender hatred or prejudice" within the preceding 12 months. Some communities also hold "Transgender Day of Recognition (TDOR)" or "Transgender Day of Visibility," or other more upbeat themes, because with the increasing numbers of transgender people killed around the world, the traditional TDOR can be very emotional, even depressing or frightening for some individuals.
- Creating a Healthier Scotland: A Conversation & Workshop (www.scottishtrans.org/event/2292/)—Offered in Edinburgh, Glasgow, and Aberdeen as part of the "nationwide consultation run by the Scottish Government and the Scottish Transgender Alliance to find out what matters to trans people in the future of health and social care."
- Trans Community Fair at Pride Toronto (Canada) (www.pridetoronto.com/wp/wp-content/uploads/2016-05-03_Pride_Toronto_Trans_Release.pdf)—"Looking for information, connections or support within the trans community? Before, during and after the Trans* March, browse the offerings of the 2016 Trans Pride Community Fair in Allan Gardens, supported and run by the fabulous and inclusive trans organizations from across the Greater Toronto Area."

Finding Support Communities for Transgender Clients

In some cities, LGBT community centers and LGBT-focused public health clinics have played a large part in providing transgender health, along with providing peer support groups for transgender people, job training programs, and social events. American cities with LGBT community centers (www.lgbtcenters.org) with transgender-focused clinics and programs include Albuquerque, NM; Atlanta, GA; Boston, MA; Dallas, TX; Denver, CO; Las Vegas, NV; Los Angeles, CA; Miami/Fort Lauderdale, FL; Missoula, MT; New York, NY; San Diego, CA: San Francisco, CA; Seattle, WA; Tucson, AZ; and Washington, DC. Cities outside of the U.S. with vibrant transgender-focused programs and clinics include Guelph, Toronto, Vancouver, and Winnipeg in Canada (www.trans-health.com/clinics); Leeds, London, Manchester, Newcastle, and Northamptonshire in England (www.nhs.uk/Livewell/Transhealth); and several other locations.

But what about those trans-identified clients who do not identify or relate to the LGBT world?

Online resources offer transgender clients valuable peer-based support and information in contexts where they don't have to be visible to others, or where they can find groups that are not overly focused on LGB or "queer" culture at the expense of a focus on transgender issues in general. For some transgender people, groups that focus on sexual orientation (even though they may welcome transgender people) can minimize or unconsciously discourage gender identity issues. Sometimes there are challenges created by different terminologies used by transgender people that are confusing or off-putting to lesbian and gay people. And transgender people may encounter internal challenges over their own sexual orientation identification as their hormonal transition progresses. However, exposure to a wider circle of potential friends can be a positive learning experience in which stereotypes can be overcome and real personal growth can occur. Here are some sources for locating community groups, and more information:

- Transgender Specific National/Statewide Activist Organizations List (U.S.)—www.masstpc.org/mediawiki/index.php?title=Transgender_Specific_National/Statewide_Activist_Organizations
- The Gender Centre, Inc (AUS)—https://gendercentre.org.au
- Trans Equality Rights in Canada—https://www.transequalitycanada.com/
- The Scottish Transgender Alliance—www.scottishtrans.org
- The Gender Trust (U.K.)—http://gendertrust.org.uk
- Transgender Europe—http://tgeu.org/

There are numerous transgender-related groups on Facebook, many of which are private, but are possible to join by submitting a request to the moderator. Encourage your clients to shop around for groups that feel comfortable and helpful to them and remind them not to believe everything they read or see on the Internet. Everyone should be able to find a corroborating, reliable source (or more than one!) for information they are not sure about; and if they cannot find corroboration then the original information should be regarded with caution until it can be verified.

Staying Up to Date on Transgender Care and Scholarship

So much is happening today in transgender health that it can be difficult to keep up with new developments. In addition to participating in a peer professional network, you may want to subscribe or monitor both professional and academic journals, depending on your interests. Also, making use of the increasingly available continuing education that is available in classroom settings or online is an excellent way to remain current, as well as develop new peer resources. Below are useful resources.

Journals

- *Transgender Health* (http://online.liebertpub.com/trgh)
- *International Journal of Transgenderism* (www.tandfonline.com/loi/wijt20)
- *Psychology of Sexual Orientation and Gender Diversity* (www.apa.org/pubs/journals/sgd)

- *LGBT Health* (www.liebertpub.com/lgbt)
- *Archives of Sexual Behavior* (http://link.springer.com/journal/10508)
- *Journal of Sex Research* (www.tandfonline.com/loi/hjsr20)
- *TSQ: Transgender Studies Quarterly* (http://tsq.dukejournals.org)

Continuing Education

- WPATH Global Education Initiative (GEI) Training and Certification Programs (www.wpath.org), offers courses in a variety of locations.
- National LGBT Health Education Center, a program of the Fenway Institute, offers two sources for transgender medical and behavioral health utilizing video conferencing, webinars, online learning modules, and training series approaches:
  - *Trans Talks* (www.lgbthealtheducation.org/topic/transgender-health/)
  - Transgender Health ECHO (www.lgbthealtheducation.org/transecho/)
- *Foundations for Psychological Practice with Transgender & Gender Nonconforming (TGNC) Clients* (www.apa.org/education/ce/pdp0013.aspx) is an American Psychological Association video on-demand CEU course that "provides basic information about trans-affirmative approaches to research, supervision and clinical work."
- U.S. Department of Veterans Affairs (VA), Veterans Health Administration (VHA), LGBT Health Program (www.patientcare.va.gov/LGBT/LGBT_Veteran_Training.asp)—"Provides ongoing educational programs for VHA staff about best practices in LGBT healthcare. Three modules on Transgender health are available on-demand outside the VA." VHA TRAIN (https://www.train.org/vha/welcome) is a free service of Public Health Foundation and operates through collaborative partnerships with state and federal agencies, local and national organizations, and educational institutions.

Connecting with Transgender Advocacy Organizations

Advocacy organizations can be extremely useful in helping you or your clients answer questions about legal or policy matters, including identity documents, foreign travel/immigration, human and civil rights with respect to interpersonal disputes (i.e., relationship dissolution, child custody), employment discrimination, school policies, freedom from bullying, and incarceration issues. Advocacy groups can also sometimes help transgender people make contact with local peer support groups, and medical resources, as well. Find these and other organizations online, and sign up for their mailing lists. You will receive periodic updates that will allow you to see regularly what the pressing issues are for the transgender community, some of which may affect your transgender clients, even if they are not connected with community organizations themselves. Here are a few suggestions to get you started:

- National Center for Transgender Equality (U.S.)—www.transequality.org
- Press for Change (U.K.)—www.pfc.org.uk/
- Centre for Gender Advocacy (Quebec, Canada)—http://genderadvocacy.org
- Trans Alliance Society (British Columbia, Canada)—www.transalliancesociety.org
- Gender Identity Australia—www.genderidentityaustralia.com
- Transgender, Gender Variant & Intersex Justice Project (U.S.)—www.tgijp.org

Conclusion

There is no reason for mental health professionals to feel isolated as they learn (more) about transgender health and how to best help their clients. Resources can readily be found on the Internet, and we have provided numerous examples, each of which will generate leads to additional resources. However, information and opportunities for professional education on transgender care are increasing at a remarkable rate, making it difficult to keep pace with the most current scholarship, changing standards and best practices, and an evolving transgender community. It can sometimes seem overwhelming to identify accurate information. This chapter provides general guidelines for locating relevant, reliable resources, and for connecting with professional peers.

Take Home Points

- Professional associations provide helpful networking and can quickly lead to practical and reliable clinical information.
- The Internet makes finding local and regional resources very easy.
- Support communities for clients can be found online and in most major cities.

Recommended Reading

To wrap up, we recommend the nine documents below as the core of your transgender resource library. Most are free downloadable documents. Not all of them will be relevant given your location or clinical focus, but each is foundational and, like everything else, can also lead you to additional resources.

- American Psychological Association's *Guidelines for Psychological Practice with Transgender and Gender Nonconforming People* (U.S.)—www.apa.org/practice/guidelines/transgender.pdf
- Association for Lesbian, Gay, Bisexual, and Transgender Issues in Counseling's (U.S.) *Competencies for Counseling Transgender Clients*—www.algbtic.org/competencies.html
- *Trans Bodies, Trans Selves: A Resource for the Trans Community* (U.S.)—http://transbodies.com
- *The Teaching Transgender Toolkit: A Facilitator's Guide to Increasing Knowledge, Decreasing Prejudice & Building Skills*—www.teachingtransgender.org/
- Royal College of Psychiatrists' *Good Practice Guidelines for the Assessment and Treatment of Adults with Gender Dysphoria* (UK)—www.rcpsych.ac.uk/files/pdfversion/CR181_Nov15.pdf
- Sherbourne Health Centre's *Guidelines and Protocol for Trans Care* (Canada) http://sherbourne.on.ca/lgbt-health/guidelines-protocols-for-trans-care
- Shipherd, J. C. (2015). Defining competence when working with sexual and gender minority populations: Training models for professional development. *Clinical Psychology: Science and Practice, 22*(2), 101–104.
- Matza, A. R., Sloan, C. A., & Kauth, M. R. (2015). Quality LGBT health education: A review of key reports and webinars. *Clinical Psychology: Science and Practice, 22*(2), 127–144.
- World Professional Association for Transgender Health, *Standards of Care for the Health of Transsexual, Transgender, and Gender-Nonconforming People, Version* 7. (2011). Retrieved from https://s3.amazonaws.com/amo_hub_content/Association140/files/Standards%20of%20Care%20V7%20-%202011%20WPATH%20(2)(1).pdf

References

World Professional Association for Transgender Health, *Standards of Care for the Health of Transsexual, Transgender, and Gender-Nonconforming People, Version* 7. (2011). Retrieved from https://s3.amazonaws.com/amo_hub_content/Association140/files/Standards%20of%20Care%20V7%20-%202011%20WPATH%20(2)(1).pdf

World Professional Association for Transgender Health. (2016). Membership statistics from the WPATH Executive Director's report to the membership at the 24th Biennial Symposium, Amsterdam, Netherlands, June 21, 2016.

13 Sexual Health Among Transgender People

Ladawn Sheffield, MA, LMHC
Alex S. Keuroghlian, MD, MPH

Transgender clients, like many people seeking mental health services, have concerns about sexual relationships, sexual health, and sexual functioning. Daskalakis, Radix, and Mayer (2015) assert that exploring sexual health with lesbian, gay, bisexual, transgender, and queer clients "requires an open-ended approach free of assumptions and judgments of how desire and sexuality can or should be expressed" (p. 290). Similar to the stance taken by Day-Vines and colleagues (2007), regarding how to discuss issues of race in the therapeutic relationship, we assert that the onus of responsibility is on the provider to broach topics of sexuality, "otherwise such dialogues might remain unexamined, reflecting in large measure the taboo nature" of sexuality in our culture (p. 402). (Healthcare professionals avoid conversations about sexuality with transgender clients out of fear of offending, inadequate training, worry about identifying problems that the provider does not know how to treat, or discomfort talking about sex generally and particularly within the context of queer identities [Daskalakis, Radix, & Mayer, 2015]). Healthcare professionals may also struggle with understanding the interplay between gender and sexuality. Not broaching sexuality with transgender clients risks perpetuating the implicit shame and invisibility surrounding transgender sexual identities.

Existing research on sexual health among transgender populations offers a limited focus, mainly exploring sexual functioning after *medical affirmation* (i.e., hormone therapy or gender-affirming surgeries) and increased risk of sexually transmitted infections (Bauer & Hammond, 2015) or perceived paraphilia (Pfeffer, 2014). This chapter utilizes research as well as clinical experience to outline therapeutic considerations for sexual health among transgender clients, including sexual identities and fluidity, sexual satisfaction, and relational health. Attention is given to providing a transgender-affirming frame and discussing sexual health risk within the context of psychosocial stressors, including gender dysphoria and experiences of transphobia. Engaging transgender clients in exploring sexuality—including intersectionality with gender identity and shifts in attraction associated with medical affirmation—is integral to the larger clinical goal of affirming transgender identities and providing competent care.

Gender and Sexuality

Sexual orientation, gender identity, and biological sex are routinely conflated in psychological and medical discourse, making it difficult to understand the sexuality of transgender clients (Bauer & Hammond, 2015; Keatley, Deutsch, Sevelius, & Gutierrez-Mock, 2015; Meier, Pardo, Labuski, & Babcock, 2013). *Sexual orientation* refers to emotional and physical attraction to people of the same and/or other genders (i.e., being lesbian, gay, bisexual, or heterosexual) (Makadon, Goldhammer, & Davis, 2015). *Gender identity* refers to a person's internal sense of their own gender (i.e., being female, male, genderqueer, or non-binary; Keatley et al., 2015). *Non-binary* and *genderqueer* can be understood to reflect identifying as neither male nor female, or identifying as both, and may reflect fluidity in gender identity. *Sex* refers to biological markers and anatomic characteristics including organs and genitalia (Keatley et al., 2015). We are assigned one of two sexes at birth, male or female, even when characteristics of both sexes are present (Keatley et al., 2015).

When understood as unchanging concepts, sexual orientation, gender identity, and sex increasingly fail to reflect the fluidity of sexual experience of transgender clients (Meier, Pardo, Labuski, & Babcock, 2013). Historically, mental health professionals acted as "gate keepers," viewing sexual orientation as an ineligibility factor for clients seeking medical affirmation since "true transgender" clients were assumed to be heterosexual (Rowniak & Chesla, 2013). It is imperative to disregard the notion of an essential or causal link between gender identity and sexual orientation (Bauer & Hammond, 2015) and instead acknowledge the mutually influencing and reinforcing nature of these discrete categories (Pfeffer, 2014; Schleifer, 2006).

Contrary to previous conceptions of sexual orientation—as a fundamental, fixed aspect of personality, formed by prenatal and early developmental factors—research indicates shifts in sexual orientation are common among transgender adults following medical gender affirmation (Bockting, Benner, & Coleman, 2009; Daskalos, 1998). Given that sexual orientation can be fluid and encompass three discrete components (desire, behavior, and identity), we will discuss how each component may be affected by medical affirmation. As we will discuss later in this chapter, supporting transgender clients in navigating these shifts is essential to transgender-affirming care.

Researchers typically define sexual orientation based on sex assigned at birth and genitalia, for example attributing heterosexual orientation to a transgender woman (assigned male sex at birth) who is primarily attracted to women although the transgender woman may identify as lesbian (Daskalos 1998). For the purpose of this chapter, we adopt the transgender-affirming conceptualization of sexual orientation related to gender identity (i.e., a transgender woman primarily attracted to women may identify as lesbian, regardless of medical affirmation) (Bauer & Hammond, 2015; Bockting, Benner, & Coleman, 2009; Keatley et al., 2015). *Female-to-male* (*FTM*) and *male-to-female* (*MTF*) are sometimes utilized in research to reference both sex assigned at birth and affirmed identity. We utilize the terms *transgender man* and *transgender woman* in lieu of FTM or MTF, respectively. These terms are used interchangeably with *transmasculine* and *transfeminine*, respectively, and reflect identity being different from sex assigned at birth, again regardless of medical affirmation. Our intention is that these terms be inclusive of the transgender spectrum, including non-binary clients for whom "man" or "woman" may not accurately reflect identity but are nonetheless on the transmasculine or transfeminine spectrum. We also acknowledge the limitations of language in reflecting agender clients who do not identify as masculine or feminine or non-binary clients who integrate both (Reisner et al., 2016).

Transgender Sexual Identities

Transgender people reflect the full spectrum of sexual orientation and sexual behavior (Bauer & Hammond, 2015; Keatley et al., 2015), challenging heteronormative misconceptions (i.e., presumed heterosexual identity). Transgender clients are more likely to identify as bisexual (sexual attraction to both men and women) or pansexual (attraction to all genders including non-binary genders) (Bauer & Hammond, 2015; Bockting, Benner, & Coleman, 2009). This is true across the lifespan, including for transgender elders (Cook-Daniels & Munson, 2010). Anecdotal experience in our clinical practice suggests transgender clients more frequently identify on the *asexual* spectrum (i.e., not engaging in sexual behavior) or having little or no sexual desire (Hill-Meyer & Scarborough, 2014). Additionally, clients on the autism spectrum are more likely to identify as asexual (Gilmore, Schalomon, & Smith, 2012) as well as transgender (Glidden, Bouman, Jones, & Arcelus, 2016) or use language from within the autistic community, such as *gendervague*, "a specifically neurodivergent experience of trans/gender identity" (Brown, 2016, June, 22). Although we recognize the validity of asexual identity and suggest an affirming stance, clients may benefit from further exploring the etiology of asexuality. Bauer and Hammond (2015) asserted that for some transfeminine clients, an asexual identity might reflect feeling excluded from the sphere of sexual identity due to transgender status. Transgender elders may feel further excluded from the sphere of sexual identity due to ageism. Mental health professionals working with transgender clients should become familiar with the spectrum of sexual identities in order to enable clients to explore their sexual or relational health concerns during treatment. At the same time, allowing clients to drive exploration of sexual health concerns may prevent creating an atmosphere in which clients feel they are the object of the provider's curiosity or required to educate their providers.

Developing a healthy sexual identity can be difficult for transgender clients who may not encounter images of empowered transgender sexuality. What Bauer and Hammond (2015) refer to as the ubiquitous "shemale" images in pornography, created for cisgender men, may create internal conflict among transgender women regarding limited expectations of transfeminine sexuality. Encouraging clients to utilize transgender-affirming sexual imagery that depicts healthy power dynamics may increase positive sexual self-image (Bauer & Hammond, 2015) as well as safer, more satisfying sex (Reisner, Perkovich, & Mimiaga, 2010). Pfeffer (2014) identifies a range of transgender-affirmative and community-generated resources on transgender sexuality. Hill-Meyer and Scarborough (2014) provide an in-depth discussion of boundaries and consent, contraception, and sex toys from a transgender-affirming, sex-positive stance. Both resources are included in the recommended reading section of this chapter.

Due to body-centered gender dysphoria, transgender clients may experience dissociation during sex (Hill-Meyer & Scarborough, 2014) and benefit from learning grounding skills to increase embodiment and pleasure. Doorduin and Van Berlo (2014) assert prior to affirmation, transgender people may try "diligently to meet social expectations" of others, making it "difficult to get in touch with their own (gender and sexual) wishes and boundaries" (p. 664). Finding comfortable language, specifically naming body parts and asking for what one desires, is difficult for many people and may pose a challenge for transgender clients, negatively affecting sexual satisfaction as well as safety (Reisner, Perkovich, & Mimiaga, 2010). For example, a transgender man who is not comfortable talking about his vagina may be unable to explicitly state that vaginal intercourse is not pleasurable. This may lead him to passively accept sexual behavior that is dissatisfying and may also trigger gender dysphoria. Identifying comfortable language about sexuality and preparing to use it with partners can help clients to manage anticipatory anxiety. This may be particularly salient for transgender clients who have elected not to alter sex characteristics yet desire being "seen" as their affirmed gender (i.e., a transgender man who has not had chest reconstructive surgery but wants partners to refer to his chest with masculine language; Schleifer, 2006). Exploring ways to reframe triggers for dysphoria may also be helpful. One transgender man interviewed by Schleifer (2006) discussed thinking of vaginal lubrication as "pre-come" in order to mitigate dysphoria and reclaim masculinity in his sexual experience.

Transgender Clients and Sexual Health

Exploring sexual health with transgender clients should be undertaken with the goal of providing information that both reduces risk and promotes physically and emotionally satisfying sex (Daskalakis, Radix, & Mayer, 2015). Rather than feeling overwhelmed, mental health providers should build on existing training and awareness of "men's" and "women's" sexual and relational health issues, with the addition of concerns specific to transgender clients (Bauer & Hammond, 2015). Quality care requires that the provider seek education on the topic, assess sexual health goals as part of regular intake, and only focus on sexual health and behavior to the extent that it aligns with the client's treatment goals. It is also important to understand that risk is associated with a person's behavior and their sexual partners, not their own sexual or gender identity (Daskalakis, Radix, & Mayer, 2015). Sexual risk assessment and risk reduction efforts require exploring what body parts are engaged with another's body parts and what fluids are exchanged, regardless of how the client or partner(s) identify themselves. For example, research indicates transgender women are disproportionately affected by HIV when having receptive, penetrative intercourse with cisgender men (Grant et al., 2016).

Assumptions and misinformation on the part of clients and providers can lead to over-looking risk. The heteronormative assumption that transgender men are only sexually active with cisgender women may lead to providers underestimating risk for *sexually transmitted infections (STIs*; Reisner, Perkovich, & Mimiaga, 2010) as well as unplanned pregnancy. Light and colleagues (2014) note that transgender men who became pregnant reported unintended pregnancy rates comparable to cisgender women. As noted by Herbst and colleagues (2008), transgender populations reported significantly higher rates of HIV infection than general populations and believed they were not at risk for HIV infection despite engaging in frequent, high-risk behavior. Additional psychosocial stressors that increase risk were identified, including mental health problems, physical abuse, social isolation, economic marginalization, and incarceration. In addition, transgender men may engage in high-risk behavior due to wanting to "belong" in gay male communities, including HIV positive circles (Rowniak & Chesla, 2013). Internalized transphobia and anxiety about sexual performance may promote high-risk behavior due to feeling "lucky" for the attention (Reisner, Perkovich, & Mimiaga, 2010). Depression and anxiety, as well as illicit substance use to manage anticipatory anxiety related to transphobia, may contribute to high-risk sexual behavior among transgender men (Reisner, Perkovich, & Mimiaga, 2010), and while not yet studied may also be true for transgender women.

Due to a power differential, transgender clients may not feel empowered to make decisions regarding drug use, condom use, and high-risk sexual behavior, making them vulnerable to traumatic sexual experiences and STI exposure. Transactional sex may be a risk factor for HIV among both transgender men (Reisner, Perkovich, & Mimiaga, 2010) and transgender women (Grant et al., 2016). Educating clients about *pre-exposure prophylaxis (PrEP)* for HIV is an effective harm reduction approach that acknowledges both risk and power differential. Research indicates high efficacy for exposure during vaginal or anal intercourse however; no studies have assessed efficacy with transgender men or with transgender women with neovaginas (Grant et al., 2016). Research indicates transfeminine clients are more likely to adhere to PrEP if prescribed by the primary care provider who also prescribes gender-affirming hormone therapy (Grant et al., 2016). Thus, connecting clients to transgender-affirming medical care may also support sexual health.

As a result of assumed heterosexual behavior, little research has been done to understand the risk for HIV and other STIs among transgender men who have sex with men (Reisner, Perkovich, & Mimiaga, 2010). Due to the potential for fluidity of sexual behavior among transgender men and shifts in sexual attractions that can occur during medical affirmation, specific interventions to reduce sexual risk are indicated (Reisner, Perkovich, & Mimiaga, 2010). Bauer and Hammond (2015) assert that most research on risk for transgender women also assumes heterosexuality, including being the receptive partner in behavior involving penetration. Due to lack of funding, research has also focused mainly on HIV risk and prevention and has not elucidated risk for other STIs or sexual health concerns, such as fertility or pregnancy (Reisner, Perkovich, & Mimiaga, 2016).

The process of medical affirmation itself may contribute to risk. Transgender men may engage in high-risk sexual behavior and experimentation in the early stages of affirmation (Reisner, Perkovich, & Mimiaga, 2010). For example, inexperienced in the social rules of gay male dating communities, transgender men who are attracted to men may have difficulty negotiating safety or may feel pressured into high-risk behavior to prove their masculinity (Reisner, Perkovich, & Mimiaga, 2010). Likewise, transgender women who are attracted to men may have difficulty negotiating safety or feel pressured to be receptive to her partner. Encouraging clients to advocate for safety and supporting them by rehearsing the negotiation of boundaries may help to minimize sexual risk during social and medical affirmation.

Discomfort talking about sexual behavior, believing that medical providers may not be knowledgeable about transgender bodies (Reisner, Perkovich, & Mimiaga, 2010), and poor treatment in gender segregated health care settings (Cook-Daniels, 2006) may prevent transgender clients from getting appropriate STI screening and care. This fear of poor or hostile treatment is particulary salient for elder transgender clients as medical issues increase with age, requiring more frequent interaction with medical providers (Cook-Daniels, 2006). Further, gender dysphoria related to primary and secondary sex characteristics may lead clients to neglect regular check-ups. The "if you have it, check it" approach to cervical cancer screenings reminds transgender men to maintain regular sexual health screenings with medical providers (Bernstein, Potter, & Peitzmeier, 2014). The same approach will also benefit transgender women regarding prostate health. Exploring why transgender clients avoid health screenings will allow mental health providers to support them in preparing for medical appointments, whether by reality testing around the need for regular screening or teaching grounding techniques to manage anxiety related to attending the appointment.

Changes in Libido and Sexual Orientation after Medical Affirmation

It is important to note that not all transgender clients desire medical affirmation. For transgender clients who do access medical affirmation, it can be helpful to forecast changes, as they may vary from gradual to sudden and unanticipated (Rowniak & Chesla, 2013). For example, transmasculine clients may experience distress related to increased libido or enjoyment of pornographic images and come to appointments asking, "Is this normal?" Transmasculine elders, for instance, starting hormone therapy in their 60s may find increased libido disruptive within an established relationship.

Research indicates hormone therapy affects libido in transgender people (Van Goozen, Cohen-Kettenis, Gooren, Frijda, & Van De Poll, 1995; Weirckx et al., 2011a). Transgender men overwhelmingly report increased libido (Bockting, Benner, & Coleman, 2009), but research is less conclusive regarding shifts in libido for transgender women. As articulated by Wierckx and colleagues (2011b), transgender men who have undergone medical affirmation experience higher frequency and intensity of sexual desire than transgender women, similar to documented disparity between cisgender men and women. Higher levels of androgens are thought to account for this disparity, along with psychological and sociocultural factors. Increased sexual desire may result from reduced gender dysphoria (Wierckx et al., 2011b) and related increased sense of embodiment. Some studies have reported decreased sexual arousal for transgender women on hormone therapy but clarify that the level of libido is not significantly different from that reported by cisgender women (Klein & Gorzalka, 2009). Other research has noted an eventual return of desire in transgender women after acclimating to hormone therapy (Doorduin & Van Berlo, 2014) or potential increase in libido related to breast development and positive mental health effects (Bauer & Hammond, 2015). It is important to note that while hormone therapy may alleviate gender dysphoria it may also inadvertently reinforce the privileging of the body as signifier of gender (i.e., having a hairy, masculinized body or breast development is "proof" of gender identity; Edelman, 2016).

Research measuring libido in transgender women may erroneously assume that loss of erectile function is desired, which complicates the relationship between this common effect of hormone therapy and satisfaction (Bauer & Hammond, 2015). Unless they are hoping to engage in penetrative sex with their penis, decrease in capacity to maintain an erection may not be troubling to transgender women as they may still experience orgasm and pleasure (Deutsch, 2014). If transgender women are sexually dissatisfied due to loss of erection, you can encourage them to speak to medical providers about adjusting their hormone regimen and/or supplementation with medications like sildenafil. Likewise, you can encourage transmasculine clients to discuss their hormone regimen with their prescriber if they are uncomfortable with increased libido.

In our clinical work we have observed increased comfort in sexual relationships after medical affirmation, likely related to alignment of identity and body. We have also witnessed the opposite, a decrease in desire and impulse to retreat from intimacy while clients acclimate to changes associated with medical affirmation. Clients may experience decreased libido but not decreased desire for intimacy or may find that what they originally thought was decreased libido was a period of adjusting to different ways of feeling desire (Hill-Meyer & Scarborough, 2014). Clients may experience orgasm differently or enjoy new types of stimulation (Hill-Meyer & Scarborough, 2014). It is important to normalize this process and support clients while they adjust to these changes.

Medical affirmation may also affect sexual orientation (Daskalos, 1998; Reisner, Perkovich, & Mimiaga, 2010), although it is unclear whether this is better attributed to increased comfort expressing other sexual attractions once gender is affirmed and body comfort is increased (Bauer & Hammond, 2015; Reisner, Perkovich, & Mimiaga, 2010). Rowniak and Chesla (2013) identify testosterone as a significant factor in a shift toward attraction to males among transgender men. Meier, Pardo, Labuski, and Babcock (2013) found that transgender men who reported exclusive attraction to women prior to medical affirmation are significantly more likely to experience attraction to men after medical affirmation. Whether this is a true shift in orientation or simply the emergence of existing desire, no longer "forbidden" in a heteronormative culture, is unclear. Similarly, transgender women may be more likely to identify as lesbian after starting hormone therapy (Bauer & Hammond, 2015). Prior to medical affirmation, body-focused gender dysphoria may be so severe as to render sexual activity impossible (Rowniak & Chesla, 2013), complicating reports of "shifts" in orientation after hormone therapy.

Transgender women have cited pressure to conform to traditional gender roles as contributing to heterosexual identity prior to medical affirmation (Daskalos, 1998). They also reported a desire to explore their emerging female gender identity through intimate connection with women, which promoted heterosexual relationships. As female identity is affirmed, transgender women may also feel free to explore and express previously repressed attractions to cisgender men (Daskalos, 1998). A similar shift may occur for transgender men. Transgender men previously attracted to cisgender men, but not acting on this attraction, may be more open to exploring this attraction once gender identity is aligned with their new masculine gender role (Reisner, Perkovich, & Mimiaga, 2010) and they are no longer seen as feminine (Schleifer, 2006). They may also become more comfortable with vaginal intercourse (Bockting, Benner, & Coleman, 2009).

Social affirmation may also alter the experience of familiar sexual behavior, within the context of shifting gender roles (Bauer & Hammond, 2015). Bauer and Hammond (2015) give the example of a transgender woman who has not had genital surgery engaging in familiar sexual behavior, like penetrative intercourse with her penis. Within the context of a lesbian relationship this act may be more similar to lesbian kink, "akin to cis[gender] lesbians using strap-ons," than penetrative intercourse within a heterosexual relationship (p. 5). Mental health professionals can forecast these possible changes for clients during therapy in order to normalize the process and alleviate distress.

Sexual Satisfaction and Gender Affirming Surgeries

Wierckx and colleagues (2011b) and Weyers et al. (2009) provide excellent summaries of gender-affirming surgeries for transgender men and transgender women, respectively, including information about techniques and complications. Chapter 9 in this book also offers a useful summary. Research is limited and divided regarding sexual satisfaction after gender-affirming surgeries: some studies indicate adequate-to-high levels of sexual satisfaction and functioning (Bockting, Benner, & Coleman, 2009; Wierckx et al., 2011b), whereas others find mixed or suboptimal satisfaction, specifically among transgender women (Bauer & Hammond, 2015; Weyers et al., 2009). Transgender clients may need time to adjust to changes in sexual functioning and physical sensitivity after surgery (Doorduin & Van Berlo, 2014), but research indicates high rates of ability to orgasm (Klein & Gorzalka, 2009).

Some transgender men desire surgery primarily to affirm gender identity, despite the functional limitations of phalloplasty (Bockting, Benner, & Coleman, 2009). Others may benefit from processing potential disappointment related to the inability to penetrate and decreased sensitivity (Doorduin & Van Berlo, 2014). Most vaginoplasties do not result in self-lubricating neo-vaginas and, if uneducated about this, transgender women may underestimate the need for lubrication (Hill-Meyer & Scarborough, 2014). Due to numerous barriers, including financial obstacles and contraindication related to age or co-occurring medical problems, many transgender clients are not able to have genital surgery (Bauer & Hammond, 2015; Meier, Pardo, Labuski, & Babcock, 2013). Medical affirmation later in life may result in less satisfactory outcomes due to age-related medical complications as well as frustration regarding exploration of sexual identity with a body that has limited strength and stamina. As mental health professionals, we can help transgender clients explore dissatisfaction with gender affirming surgeries, as well as frustration regarding lack of access. We can also normalize challenges with sexual functioning and support clients in developing a more positive relationship with their bodies.

Edelman and Zimman (2014) explore the ways in which transgender men who have not undergone surgical affirmation use language and metaphor to reframe their bodies as desirable within gay sexual experiences. Rather than focus on perceived lack of desirable "male" genitalia, transgender men reframe vaginas as a "bonus hole" providing greater flexibility and sexual desirability (Edelman & Zimman, 2014). Counter to the "born in the wrong body" narrative that implicitly encourages transgender clients to seek medical remedies, this reframing offers an opportunity to explore sexual satisfaction within the existing body and clarifies the distinction between biological sex characteristics and gender, "suggesting that sex is, in fact, open to self-determination such that a 'male body' can be defined as the body of a (self-identified) man" (Edelman & Zimman, 2014).

Relational Health

It would be a mistake to minimize the difficulty transgender clients may experience in seeking sexual and romantic partners. Adopting the stance that "dating is hard for everyone" is invalidating and does not acknowledge cisgender privilege. Research suggests transgender women may fear rejection and thus delay disclosing their transgender status, which may greatly diminish opportunities for emotional and sexual intimacy (Daskalos, 1998), and this is likely also true for transgender men. Transgender clients may also fear violence related to transphobia or homophobia upon disclosing their transgender status. Partners may pressure transgender clients to undergo, or conversely to delay, gender-affirming surgery. Relative invisibility for transgender men who are on hormones and "pass" may add to difficulty disclosing transgender status (Bockting, Benner, & Coleman, 2009). In *Trans Bodies, Trans Selves: A Resource for the Transgender Community*, Hill-Meyer and Scarborough (2014) provide a thoughtful synopsis of the complexity of deciding when and how to disclose transgender status to potential partners. While we can support clients in exploring hopes and fears related to disclosure, providing peer generated resources like *Trans Bodies, Trans Selves* and encouraging them to seek out peer support groups will normalize the process.

Due to the pervasive stereotype of transgender women as sex workers, transfeminine clients may be fetishized by potential suitors and find themselves the object of sexual desire but not the recipients of relational or emotional security (Bauer & Hammond, 2015). Transmasculine clients may fear being abandoned for "real men," possessing sexual characteristics unattainable through medical affirmation. Transgender elders who undergo gender affirmation later in life may struggle with feeling "out of step" with peers in sexual identity exploration and development. Acknowledging these distinct challenges and supporting clients in seeking safe, fulfilling relationships is integral to supporting mental and sexual health.

Shifts in sexual attraction and desire can put considerable strain on relationships (Bauer & Hammond, 2015), and it may be appropriate to refer clients and their partners to couples counseling that is inclusive of sexual issues or encourage cisgender partners of transgender clients to seek therapeutic support. The gender affirmation of one partner changes the public representation of the couple (i.e., a couple that was previously viewed as lesbian or gay may now be "read" as heterosexual; Bauer & Hammond, 2015), which may be uncomfortable for queer-identified clients or their partners. If a longstanding relationship dissolves due to gender affirmation later in life, elder transgender clients may face the difficult task of dating for the first time in decades (Cook-Daniels, 2006). Due to generational differences, transgender elders may face increased transphobia when seeking age-matched partners.

Medical affirmation and subsequent shifts in sexual orientation may also result in loss of community support. Transgender men attracted to women may struggle to find acceptance, and potential partners, within a previously supportive lesbian community (Meier, Pardo, Labuski, & Babcock, 2013). This may be a profound loss given the high number of transgender men who previously identified as lesbian at some point in their identity development (Bockting, Benner, & Coleman, 2009). Many transgender men may identify as queer rather than heterosexual, despite exclusive attraction to women, due to discomfort with a heteronormative identity (Rowniak & Chesla, 2013). Due to historic tension between feminist and lesbian communities and transgender communities, transgender men seeking relationships within lesbian communities may encounter transphobia (Rowniak & Chesla, 2013). Cook-Daniels (2006) notes that elder lesbians may not consider dating transgender women and cited "several older lesbian dating email lists" that "refuse to accept MTF members" (p. 23). Transgender elders are significantly less likely to identify as queer (Cook-Daniels & Munson, 2010) and may therefore feel uncomfortable in "queer" spaces or with the language more commonly used among younger transgender adults. Transgender men attracted to men may similarly face rejection within the gay community, particularly if they elect not to have genital surgery (Meier, Pardo, Labuski, & Babcock, 2013). This rejection, echoed in internalized transphobia and gender dysphoria, may inhibit sexual identity development.

Encouraging transgender clients to engage with community support can promote both relational health and sexual identity development. Fostering hope in relational goals is also essential. In a study of transgender men by Bockting and colleagues (2009), 40% reported success in maintaining sexually and emotionally fulfilling relationships, similar to reported success of gay/bisexual cisgender men in the comparison group. In a survey of transgender adults over age 50, 36% reported being in a committed or long-term relationship, and 14% were legally married (Cooke-Daniels & Munson, 2010). Transgender clients may resist connecting with transgender communities, due to internalized transphobia or a desire to blend; however, research (Bockting, Benner, & Coleman, 2009) and anecdotal experience suggest transgender clients find the greatest support and permission to explore sexual identity among transgender peers.

Take Home Points

Supporting transgender clients in exploring sexuality and improving sexual health is an essential component of transgender-affirming clinical care. Providers should strive to:

- Adopt an open and affirming stance when exploring sexual identity and health
- Acknowledge the complexity and interplay of sexual identity, gender, and sex
- Discern risk based on behavior, not identity, when promoting safe sex practices

- Self-educate about sexual identities and transgender-affirming resources
- Encourage clients to maintain sexual health care, including regular screenings
- Teach grounding skills to manage gender dysphoria and increase embodiment
- Forecast potential changes in libido and sexual satisfaction related to medical affirmation
- Normalize shifts in sexual attraction and the unique challenges of dating
- Support clients in reframing and naming body parts to increase sexual satisfaction
- Encourage clients to engage in peer supports and utilize peer-created resources

Recommended reading

Erickson-Schroth, L. (Ed.). (2014). *Trans bodies, trans selves: A resource for the transgender community*. New York, NY: Oxford University Press.

Makadon, H. J., Mayer, K. H., Potter, J., & Goldhammer, H. (Eds.). *Fenway guide to lesbian, gay, bisexual, and transgender health, 2nd edition*. Philadelphia, PA: ACP Press.

Trans Sexualities [Special Issue] (2014). *Journal of Homosexuality, 61*(5).

References

Bauer, G. R., & Hammond, R. (2015). Toward a broader conceptualization of trans women's sexual health. *The Canadian Journal of Human Sexuality, 24*(1), 1–11.

Bernstein, I., Potter, J., & Peitzmeier, S. M. (2014). If you have it, check it: overcoming barriers to cervical cancer screening with patients on the female-to-male transgender spectrum. Retrieved from www.lgbthealtheducation.org/wp-content/uploads/Overcoming-Barriers-to-Cervical-Cancer-Screening.pdf

Bockting, W., Benner, A., & Coleman, E. (2009). Gay and bisexual identity development among female-to-male transsexuals in North America: Emergence of a transgender sexuality. *Archives of Sexual Behavior, 38*(5), 688–701.

Brown, L. (2016, June, 22). Gendervague: at the intersection of Autistic and trans experiences [web log post]. Retrieved from https://thetaskforceblog.org/2016/06/22/gendervague-at-the-intersection-of-autistic-and-trans-experiences/

Cook-Daniels, L. (2006). Trans aging. In D. Kimmel, T. Rose, & S. David (Eds.), *Lesbian, gay, bisexual and transgender aging: Research and clinical perspectives* (pp. 20–35). New York, NY: Columbia University.

Cook-Daniels, L., & Munson, M. (2010). Sexual violence, elder abuse, and sexuality of transgender adults, age 50+: Results of three surveys. *Journal of GLBT Family Studies, 6*(2), 142–177.

Daskalakis, D., Radix, A., Mayer, G. (2015). Sexual health of LGBTQ people. In H. J. Makadon, K. H. Mayer, J. Potter, & H. Goldhammer (Eds.), *The Fenway guide to lesbian, gay, bisexual, and transgender health, 2nd edition* (pp. 289–324). Philadelphia, PA: ACP Press.

Daskalos, C. T. (1998). Changes in the sexual orientation of six heterosexual male-to-female transsexuals. *Archives of Sexual Behavior, 27*(6), 605–614.

Day-Vines, N. L., Wood, S. M., Grothaus, T., Craigen, L., Holman, A., Dotson-Blake, K., & Douglass, M. J. (2007). Broaching the subjects of race, ethnicity, and culture during the counseling process. *Journal of Counseling and Development, 85*(4), 401.

Deutsch, M. (2014). Medical Transition. In L. Schroth (Ed.), *Trans bodies, trans selves: A resource for the transgender community* (pp 241–264). New York, NY: Oxford University.

Doorduin, T., & Van Berlo, W. (2014). Trans people's experience of sexuality in the Netherlands: A pilot study. *Journal of Homosexuality, 61*(5), 654–672.

Edelman, E. A. (2016). "This is where you fall off my map": Trans-spectrum spatialities in Washington, DC, safety, and the refusal to submit to somatic erasure. *Journal of Homosexuality, 63*(3), 394–404.

Edelman, E. A., & Zimman, L. (2014). Boycunts and bonus holes: Trans men's bodies, neoliberalism, and the sexual productivity of genitals. *Journal of Homosexuality, 61*(5), 673–690.

Gilmore, L., Schaloman, P. M., & Smith, V. (2012). Sexuality in a community-based sample of adults with autism spectrum disorder. *Research in Autism Spectrum Disorders, 6*(1), 313–318.

Glidden, D., Bouman, W. P., Jones, B. A., & Arcelus, J. (2016). Gender dysphoria and autism spectrum disorder: A systematic review of the literature. *Sexual Medicine Reviews, 4*(1), 3–14.

Grant, R. M., Sevelius, J. M., Guanira, J.V., Aguilar, J.V., Chariyalertsak, S., & Deutsch, M. B. (2016). Transgender women in clinical trials of pre-exposure prophylaxis. *Journal of Acquired Immune Deficiency Syndromes, 72*, S226–S229.

Herbst, J. H., Jacobs, E. D., Finlayson, T. J., McKleroy, V. S., Neumann, M. S., Crepaz, N., & HIV/AIDS Prevention Research Synthesis Team. (2008). Estimating HIV prevalence and risk behaviors of transgender persons in the United States: A systematic review. *AIDS and Behavior, 12*(1), 1–17.

Hill-Meyer, T., Scarborough, D. (2014). Sexuality. In L. Schroth (Ed.), *Trans bodies, trans selves: A resource for the transgender community* (pp. 355–389). New York, NY: Oxford University.

Keatley, J., Deutsch, M., Sevelius, J., Gutierrez-Mock, L. (2015). Creating a foundation for improving trans health: Understanding trans identities and health care needs. In H. J. Makadon, K. H. Mayer, J. Potter, & H. Goldhammer (Eds.), *The Fenway guide to lesbian, gay, bisexual, and transgender health, 2nd edition* (pp. 459–478). Philadelphia, PA: ACP Press.

Klein, C., & Gorzalka, B. B. (2009). Continuing Medical Education: Sexual functioning in transsexuals following hormone therapy and genital surgery: A review (CME). *The Journal of Sexual Medicine, 6*(11), 2922–2939.

Light, A. D., Obedin-Maliver, J., Sevelius, J. M., & Kerns, J. L. (2014). Transgender men who experienced pregnancy after female-to-male gender transitioning. *Obstetrics & Gynecology, 124*(6), 1120–1127.

Makadon, H. J., Goldhammer, H., Davis, J. (2015). Providing optimal health care for LGBT people: Changing the clinical environment and educating professionals. In H. J. Makadon, K. H. Mayer, J. Potter, & H. Goldhammer (Eds.), *The Fenway guide to lesbian, gay, bisexual, and transgender health, 2nd edition* (pp. 3–21). Philadelphia, PA: ACP Press.

Meier, S. C., Pardo, S. T., Labuski, C., & Babcock, J. (2013). Measures of clinical health among female-to-male transgender persons as a function of sexual orientation. *Archives of Sexual Behavior, 42*(3), 463–474.

Pfeffer, C. A. (2014). Making space for trans sexualities. *Journal of Homosexuality, 61*(5), 597–604.

Reisner, S. L., Perkovich, B., & Mimiaga, M. J. (2010). A mixed methods study of the sexual health needs of New England transmen who have sex with nontransgender men. *AIDS Patient Care and STDs, 24*(8), 501–513.

Reisner, S. L., Poteat, T., Keatley, J., Cabral, M., Mothopeng, T., Dunham, E., Holland, C. E., Max, R., Baral, S. D. (2016). Global health burden and needs of transgender populations: A review. *The Lancet, 388* (10042), 412–436.

Rowniak, S., & Chesla, C. (2013). Coming out for a third time: Transmen, sexual orientation, and identity. *Archives of Sexual Behavior, 42*(3), 449–461.

Schleifer, D. (2006). Make me feel mighty real: Gay female-to-male transgenderists negotiating sex, gender, and sexuality. *Sexualities, 9*(1), 57–75.

Van Goozen, S. H., Cohen-Kettenis, P. T., Gooren, L. J., Frijda, N. H., & Van De Poll, N. E. (1995). Gender differences in behaviour: Activating effects of cross-sex hormones. *Psychoneuroendocrinology, 20*(4), 343–363.

Wierckx, K., Elaut, E., Van Caenegem, E., Van De Peer, F., Dedecker, D., Van Houdenhove, E., & T'Sjoen, G. (2011b). Sexual desire in female-to-male transsexual persons: Exploration of the role of testosterone administration. *European Journal of Endocrinology, 165*(2), 331–337.

Wierckx, K., Van Caenegem, E., Elaut, E., Dedecker, D., Van de Peer, F., Toye, K. & T'Sjoen, G. (2011a). Quality of life and sexual health after sex reassignment surgery in transsexual men. *Journal of Sexual Medicine, 8*(12), 3379–3388.

Weyers, S., Elaut, E., De Sutter, P., Gerris, J., T'Sjoen, G., Heylens, G., De Cuypere, G., & Verstraelen, H. (2009). Long-term assessment of the physical, mental, and sexual health among transsexual women. *Journal of Sexual Medicine, 6*(3), 752–760.

14 Implementing a Transgender Care Policy in a National Healthcare System

Jillian C. Shipherd, PhD
Michael R. Kauth, PhD
George R. Brown, MD, DFAPA

The views expressed in this material are those of the authors and do not reflect the official policy or position of the Department of Veterans Affairs or the U.S. Government.

People may be surprised to learn that the United States (U.S.) Department of Veterans Affairs' Veterans Health Administration (VHA) has been treating transgender veterans for decades (e.g., Brown, 1988). Likely it is surprising because the U.S. military had policies that explicitly prevented transgender people from serving openly until the summer of 2016 (Cronk, 2016). Just like with other people who join the military, the reasons why transgender people join the U.S. military are varied and individualized. These reasons are more complex when bans on open service are in place. However, it is clear that transgender people have served in the U.S. military at least since the American Civil War, as the example of Albert Cashier illustrates (Gansler, 2005). Eighteen other countries, including the United Kingdom, Australia, Canada, and Israel, allow transgender people to serve openly in their militaries, and the U.S. now joins their ranks (Elders et al., 2014).

In 2014, when transgender military service was still banned, the Williams Institute (an independent research center focused on sexual orientation and gender identity law and public policy) estimated that there were 134,300 transgender veterans and another 15,500 transgender people serving in the armed forces (Gates & Herman, 2014). Now that current U.S. military service members can serve openly and access transition-related care, it is expected that these numbers will rise. In addition, new enlistees may be open about transgender identities, although they will need to have completed their medical transition (individually defined) prior to joining the service. While the Department of Veterans Affairs is separate from the Department of Defense (DoD), the nearly 9 million veterans who are treated by the VHA have the common history of having served in the military during the military ban on being open about transgender identity. Given this unique context, it can be helpful to review VHA's stance toward transgender health care as there are important lessons learned that can be applied to other health care systems, especially national systems.

Overview of the U.S. Department of Veterans Affairs

The U.S. Department of Veterans Affairs houses three branches: The National Cemetery Administration (NCA), which coordinates burials, headstone markers, and medallions as well as burial flags for veterans, honors veterans and their families with final resting places in national shrines and with lasting tributes that commemorate their service and sacrifice to the country. The NCA also manages the 135 National Cemeteries (Department of Veterans Affairs, 2017a). The Veterans Benefits Administration (VBA) manages access to a variety of benefits including service-connected disability compensation, education benefits, home loan guarantees, and survivor benefits granted to family members (Department of Veterans Affairs, 2017b). Finally, the VHA is the healthcare branch, which is the largest integrated healthcare system in the U.S.

VHA has over 1,700 sites where health care is delivered and provides services to nearly 9 million veterans annually, or about a third of all living military veterans (Department of Veterans Affairs, 2017c). Veterans' eligibility to use the VHA depends on the type of their military discharge status, income, and other criteria. Eligible veterans who work may choose to use private care through non-VHA health insurance. Thus, the VHA predominantly treats veterans without private insurance and specializes in treatment of combat-related disabilities and chronic conditions, resulting in a patient population that tends to be sicker and more economically disadvantaged than other large healthcare systems (Phillips, Shahoumian, & Backus, 2015). Given the history of VHA's association with the DoD as well as the size and complexity of the VHA, it may surprise people that VHA has begun several national programs to address the needs of transgender veterans, which is the focus of this chapter.

History of VHA Transgender Care Policy

VHA providers have likely been treating transgender veterans for as long as VHA has existed, but the level of awareness and sensitivity to the concerns of transgender veteran clients has shifted over time. In the early 1990s, VHA created a Medical Benefits Package (Department of Veterans Affairs, 2016a) in order to more clearly specify included and excluded health care benefits. Among the excluded items that continue to be prohibited at VHA (nor paid for by VHA in private settings) are undefined "gender alterations". There are several reports of VHA providers who chose to interpret this exclusion narrowly (e.g., Brown, 1988; Maguen, Shipherd & Harris, 2005). However, with only the national Medical Benefits Package as guidance, there was little protection for providers offering care that could be interpreted as potentially "gender altering" such as hormone therapy and/or gender identity counseling. It was not until September 2007 that a local VHA policy (VA Boston Healthcare System Patient Care Memorandum 11-046-LM "Management of Transgender Veteran Patients"; Charness, 2011) interpreted the "gender alterations" exclusion as narrowly as possible: that is, strictly meaning surgical procedures such as chest and genital reconstruction. Other VHA facilities also began making their own local interpretation of transgender care coverage. Different local interpretations were problematic for a national healthcare system. For example, when veterans moved from one city to another, coverage for transition-related medications and therapies might have varied. For this reason, a standardization of care coverage occurred June 2011 with VHA Directive 2011-024 "Providing Health Care for Transgender and Intersex Veterans," which stated:

> It is VHA policy that medically necessary care is provided to enrolled or otherwise eligible intersex and transgender Veterans, including hormonal therapy, mental health care, preoperative evaluation, and medically necessary post-operative and long-term care following sex reassignment surgery. Sex reassignment surgery cannot be performed or funded by VHA.
>
> (p. 2)

In this way, it was possible to assure that veterans were offered treatment consistently throughout the healthcare system. Thus, with this new mandate VHA facilities were required to either provide transition-related care, or they would need to pay non-VHA providers in the community to provide this treatment. Because of this new policy, VHA facilities had an incentive to train their providers in quality transgender treatment, as this is usually less expensive than paying for community-based care.

The Directive was renewed in February 2013 with the addition of a Frequently Asked Questions (FAQ) section and remains the current policy for VHA at the time of this writing in mid-2017. The VHA directive clarified that veterans were not required to have had any specific treatment (e.g., surgical intervention) to be treated based upon their self-identified gender. Perhaps the most progressive section of the policy was as follows:

> Patients will be addressed and referred to based on their self-identified gender. Room assignments and access to any facilities for which gender is normally a consideration (e.g., restrooms) will give preference to the self-identified gender, irrespective of appearance and/or surgical history, in a manner that respects the privacy needs of transgender and non-transgender patients alike. Where there are questions or concerns related to room assignments, an ethics consultation may be requested.
>
> (p. 3)

Thus, VHA was among the first large health care organizations to assure access to bathrooms and room assignments that were consistent with the veteran's self-identified gender. Federal policies (such as this VHA directive) supersede city, town, or state ordinances that required transgender people to use bathrooms and other public accommodations consistent with their birth sex. It should also be noted that the VHA Patient Rights and Responsibilities policy (Department of Veterans Affairs, 2015) was also modified to include gender identity and expression:

> You will be treated with dignity, compassion, and respect as an individual. Consistent with Federal law, VA policy, and accreditation standards of The Joint Commission, you will not be subject to discrimination for any reason, including for reasons of age, race, ethnicity, religion, culture, language, physical or mental disability, socioeconomic status, sex, sexual orientation, or gender identity or expression.

The addition of a lengthy FAQ section to the revised Directive on transgender care provided specific answers to multiple clinical questions that had arisen after the release of the original Directive, some of which were not anticipated at the time. For example, it was not clear whether the mandated transgender healthcare policy covered electrolysis for appropriately transgender veterans. The FAQ's clarified this question (electrolysis was excluded) and many others that came from VHA clinicians. However, policies alone do not change culture and for that programmatic information and educational interventions were needed. Moreover, very few graduate training programs offer training in transgender health leading to a paucity of trained clinicians most systems (e.g., Cochran & Roboham, 2015). This deficit in training, coupled with prior VHA's limits on transgender care, meant that VHA providers were in need of education so they could offer the new required care.

VHA Transgender Care Education

Soon after publication of the transgender care Directive in 2011, a national workgroup was formed to disseminate information about this new policy. As word spread about this nationwide expectation of quality care for transgender veterans, VHA health care providers sought education, training, and clinical resources. It is worth noting that about this time the U.S. Congress repealed the law that excluded openly gay people from serving in the military which also raised concerns among providers about the health care needs of gay, lesbian, and bisexual veterans. In response, the VHA Office of Patient Care Services, the umbrella program overseeing most clinical services in VHA, formed a Lesbian, Gay, Bisexual, and Transgender (LGBT) Health Program to field questions from providers, develop education and training programs, and continue policy development to address the needs of LGBT veterans. Much of the programs and resources discussed in this chapter can be found on the VHA LGBT Health Program website (https://www.patientcare.va.gov/LGBT/).

Web-based Resources and Trainings

One of the first initiatives undertaken by the LGBT Health Program for promotion of quality transgender health within VHA was the development of an internal online resource center that could be regularly updated (although outside the scope of this chapter, a parallel processed occurred with development of an internal online resource for lesbian, gay, and bisexual veteran health). Through this website, all VHA employees can access archived presentations, journal articles, links to policies and professional society guidelines, information about support groups for veterans, awareness campaign posters, and fact sheets about transgender health. This website has become a definitive resource for VHA employees nationwide who are interested in staying abreast of the latest news and literature in transgender health. Moreover, it is an easy place to find transgender-friendly VHA-approved posters, media messages, and fact sheets for staff who want to create a welcoming environment.

Concurrent with the development of this internal VHA website, the LGBT Health Program developed three online training programs about transgender health and obtained continuing education credits for most professions. These trainings continue to be available and are located both within the VHA system through our online education platform (Talent Management System) and outside the agency through a public Internet site (VHA TRAIN https://vha.train.org/). There are a couple of compelling aspects of these trainings. First, there are several embedded videos in the trainings of vignettes where actors demonstrate culturally-competent skills. Second, and perhaps the best feature of these trainings, transgender veterans offer video testimonials about the importance of person-specific care. The first program, *An Introduction to Transgender Veteran Health Care*, is designed to improve access to respectful, top quality health care by addressing the rights of veterans to self-identify their gender for pronoun use, room assignments, and gender-based identification in the electronic medical record. The second program, *Transgender Mental Health Services*, discusses how gender transition goals vary widely among transgender people and describes the process of providing culturally-competent therapy to transgender veterans. In addition, mental health professionals are instructed in how to determine readiness to receive hormone treatments or gender confirmation surgery. The third training program, *Transgender Health: Prescribing Cross-sex Hormones*, reviews the safe and appropriate use of hormone therapy. The benefits of online trainings, like these, include being able to convey general information to a wide audience, having information available at any time, and providing continuing education credit incentives to learners. However, this format does not allow for the tailoring of general information to any one specific case, where there may be comorbidities or psychosocial challenges that complicate the clinical presentation.

Two Clinical Consultation Programs

With the collaboration of other offices within the VHA system, the LGBT Health Program has been able to offer two types of clinical consultation (transgender e-consultation and transgender team training), which allow for the tailoring of information so that the advice offered is individualized to the specific veteran's situation, including both medical and mental health comorbidities. With *transgender e-consultation*, any VHA clinician can submit a non-acute, non-urgent clinical question through the veteran's electronic health record (with the veteran's consent), and a regionally located, experienced interdisciplinary team will respond through the patient's chart within seven days (Kauth et al., 2015; Shipherd, Kauth & Matza, 2016). The benefit of this program is that the consultants can remotely review the veteran's information, including lab results, progress notes, medications, etc., before formulating a response. In some cases, the team realizes that there is a question that the provider should have asked (based on chart review) but did not ask, and they are able to provide that information too. The second clinical consultation program is *transgender team training* which is a videoconference-based course. In this seven-month long program, learner teams that include at least one mental health professional and one medical provider meet via videoconference with an interdisciplinary experienced teaching team for one hour, twice per month for a total of 14 sessions. It is worth noting that on average teams include five providers from multiple disciplines such as psychology, social work, psychiatry, endocrinology, primary care medicine, and nursing, as well as allied health professions such as speech pathology (Shipherd et al., 2016). In each session, members of the teaching team give a 15-to-20-minute didactic presentation on an aspect of transgender veteran care and then engage in case-based consultation on a case with all the participating teams at multiple sites listening to the discussion and advice on the treatment plan. Each participating team is required to present cases at some point in the seven-month course, while the other teams listen and ask questions. In this way, the participating teams learn from each other as well as from the experienced providers.

Postdoctoral Training

Across VHA there are now nine postdoctoral psychology residencies in LGBT health through the Offices of Academic Affiliations and Mental Health Services (for a list of sites, https://www.patientcare.va.gov/LGBT/LGBT_Veteran_Training.asp). While the focus is not solely on transgender health, residents are offered training in best practices in transgender veteran care and many provide direct clinical services to transgender veterans, such as gender counseling, support groups, and hormone therapy evaluations. In addition, residents provide education to both clinical and clerical staff, engage with community partners, and also spearhead local participation in national events such as the Transgender Day of Remembrance (Kauth, Shipherd, Barrera, Ortigo, & Jones, 2016).

Electronic Health Records

In addition to the clinical consultation programs described above, some additional changes are anticipated in the VHA electronic health record that will promote a more welcoming clinical environment for transgender veterans. First, in 2017 all of VA (VHA, VBA, NCA) will move to a two-step system of assessing sex and gender (Cahill & Makadon, 2014). Sex listed on the veterans' original birth certificate will assist in assuring preventive health screens (e.g., mammogram, prostate-specific antigen test) continue if a veteran has the relevant anatomy. The new self-identified gender identity demographic field that will be added to all veteran record systems will aid staff in using appropriate salutations and gender references. The second planned change to the record system, not just health records, is the addition of a preferred name field. Preferred name is relevant for all veterans as many people have nicknames or other names that they prefer to use in conversation. Someone named James John Smith may prefer to be called Jim, Jimmy, John, or go by JJ. In the case of a transgender veteran, the preference might be Jenny or another name that coincides with the veteran's gender identity. Moreover, being called into an appointment from a waiting area by one's legal name, rather than preferred name, is problematic as it violates the transgender veteran's confidentiality and "outs" them in a semi-public space, which may put them at risk for discrimination and violence. Using a transgender client's preferred name and gender identity is also respectful. In all cases (irrespective of gender identity), interactions with both clinical and clerical staff can be improved by using the client's preferred name. As patient-provider communication improves, so too will the quality of the care improve that is offered to all clients, especially for transgender clients.

Ongoing Evaluation and Improvements

Perhaps one of the most significant changes made at VHA in recent years is the appointment of LGBT Veteran Care Coordinators at every facility (Kauth & Shipherd, 2016). These "boots on the ground" champions at each facility assist VHA in addressing local veteran care needs as well as staff education gaps. LGBT Veteran Care Coordinators receive training to assure that they know about the resources described above and feel equipped to conduct local ongoing needs assessments. Part of their work is to develop local solutions for the challenges that veterans encounter at their facility. Towards this end, the LGBT Veteran Care Coordinators need to ally themselves with patient advocates, VHA police, chiefs of clinical programs, facility leadership, and LGBT Equal Employment Opportunity officers (since many veterans are both employees and clients) and ensure that key stakeholders have the relevant information to create a healthy and welcoming care environment.

As part of this effort, VHA has been participating in the Human Rights Campaign's Healthcare Equality Index (HEI) Survey (www.hrc.org/hei). The HEI Survey is a self-assessment for health care organizations to identify and close gaps in LGBT competence within an organization. For many VHA facilities, the HEI Survey has been helpful in identifying ongoing areas for growth and has offered some validation for those who were able to achieve the coveted "Leadership" status (Department of Veterans Affairs, 2016b).

Limitations of the Current State of Transgender Care at VHA

The 2011 transgender healthcare directive drove a system-wide change in attitudes and knowledge about transgender health. With a small but dedicated group of providers who were willing to provide training and offer nationwide consultation, VHA is now widely viewed as having a capacity to treat transgender veterans that far exceeds other large systems. Indeed, discussions about how to replicate our training successes in the DoD have begun. However, six years after the initial transgender care policy, VHA still faces many challenges in meeting the needs of transgender veterans. First, when the policy was initially implemented, no thought had been given to the record systems (i.e., no gender identity field, no preferred name field) and how they created barriers to providing the care that was required. Second, in 2011 few providers had any training in culturally competent transgender care and, thus, the VHA system needed to respond quickly to the demand from the field for more education and training before providers could offer this care. Third, in 2011 VHA providers were steeped in the culture of non-inclusion of transgender people that was a remnant of DoD's policies. Although DoD policy has changed, changing culture in VHA is an ongoing process, even while we offer care to several thousand transgender veterans.

Additionally, current VHA policy (i.e., the Medical Benefits Package) restricts access to services, specifically transition-related surgical procedures that are medically necessary care and increasingly covered by other types of health insurance. At the time of this writing, a VHA policy change is under review, but funding for adding gender transition surgeries has yet to be identified. Further, while the programs described above have been well received, staff participation is largely voluntary. For busy providers, this can sometimes be a challenge. As with all systems, changing the practices of disinterested or resistant staff is also challenging, but the support from VHA leadership has been helpful in addressing these challenges. Relatedly, primary care providers with no prior training in transition-related hormone treatment can be cautious about providing this service without consultation from endocrinologists. This sometimes creates a bottle-neck in services while primary care providers wait for the veteran to be seen by the specialty care service. Fortunately, the availability of clinical e-consultation programs described above is helping with this challenge. Also, the recent addition of the LGBT Veteran Care Coordinators at each facility opens opportunities for better communication and addressing providers' concerns with training.

Lessons from VHA That Can Be Applied to Other Healthcare Settings

For healthcare systems that are considering how to be responsive to transgender health needs, here are some suggestions based on our experience with the VHA. First, rather than taking a piecemeal approach, develop a strategic plan with a timeline, realizing that policy, record systems, forms, signage, outreach materials, and the physical environment of care will likely need to change (see Chapter 4 for more details). In your plan, it is important to understand that inclusive policies (e.g., non-discrimination policy) are essential but not sufficient to create cultural and practice change. Just informing staff of a policy change will not in itself lead to practice change. Funding for quality education and training and repeating the messages from these trainings are necessary for improving access to quality care for transgender people. Concurrently, identifying a motivated group of individuals with energy and authority (or access to those with authority) to enact change is key. Agency leadership must be onboard with the strategic plan and they must take it seriously. Representatives from administration and from various clinical disciplines are important to include in a strategic planning work-group. Once members are identified, formalizing and legitimizing their recommendations through the creation of an official workgroup, committee, or program can assist adoption of their recommendations. Workgroups and committees usually make initial recommendations and are time-limited; programs usually have a clear mission and a longer lifetime. Staff participating in workgroups or programs need dedicated time to complete their work. They may also find it necessary to consult with content experts on transgender care outside the agency, if that expertise does not exist locally. External expert consultants can also be of assistance in considering other perspectives on tackling difficult systems issues. The identification of content experts (internal, external, or both) who can respond to both clinical and administrative questions (e.g., preferred name and gender in the chart) that might arise is essential.

Next, the workgroup will need to identify the existing policies and procedures that apply to transgender clients (e.g., patient non-discrimination policies, room assignments, clinical reminders, record systems, billing processes) and note where changes are needed to assure that the healthcare system is inclusive and client-focused. To be a welcoming health care environment, the facility must explicitly counter the expectation of discrimination that many transgender clients have (with good reason). It is possible to do this with a combination of signage, inclusive forms, and communication of polices that are inclusive of transgender people (see Chapter 4 for additional guidance on creating a welcoming environment). Communication should make it clear what transgender clients can do when they encounter difficulties within the system and who can assist them in addressing their concerns. For example, a patient advocate can be very effective when easily accessible and on site. The workgroup may consider recommending that the agency participate in a self-study (such as the HEI Survey) to assess the system's relative strengths and weaknesses.

Given that few health care professionals have received any training in transgender care, it is highly likely that staff training will be necessary. Effective training that results in practice change needs to be provided in different formats for different types of learners as well as in different levels of knowledge because staff have different roles. In addition, training needs to be repeated and reinforced in order for new knowledge to be applied. Be sure to include non-clinical administrative staff in trainings focused on respectful communication and interactions with transgender people. The agency should utilize high quality trainings and resources on cultural and clinical competence, many of which are readily available on the Internet and at no cost (see Matza, Sloan, & Kauth, 2015). These trainings should address the intersectionality of minority identities such as sexual minority status or military veteran status (as discussed in Chapter 3). It is important to remember that making sustainable changes in a complex healthcare system is an iterative process and initial plans may not work out as intended and may need to be modified to address the context of your environment. Employing a continual quality improvement process will help committees or programs effectively implement and improve their initiatives.

Transgender cultural competence is more than a clinical skill or body of knowledge. Culturally competent care strives to create a healthcare system where all levels of care, policy, training, resources, and leadership take into account the unique needs of your transgender clients (Matza, Sloan, & Kauth, 2015). For a healthcare system to truly address transgender needs, it must continually evolve at the organizational, structural, and clinical levels. The VHA is committed to demonstrating excellence in the service of the U.S. veteran population, not only because it is the ethical and the right thing to do, but also because quality health care improves outcomes and ultimately lowers costs (Padula, Heru, & Campbell, 2016). Thus, addressing health equity, such as providing quality transgender care, makes good business sense. A fair equitable system promotes better patient engagement and better health outcomes and also supports staff who feel that they are really making a difference.

Take Home Points

- Change is always difficult, but possible no matter how large the system.
- Strategic organization and planning can assist with making comprehensive change.
- System change requires coordination of policy, procedures, and staff training.

- Consider changes to record systems that are inclusive of preferred names and pronouns.
- Task workgroups or committees with developing a strategic plan for implementing improved care for transgender clients, including periodic re-evaluation of the impact of the changes made (positive and negative) and periodically re-assess next steps.
- Making changes in a complex healthcare system can be achieved through sustained effort by champions in the system.
- If a large, complex national healthcare system like the VHA can effect change to provide culturally and clinically competent care, then smaller, simpler and more nimble systems can certainly do it!

Recommended Reading

Kauth, M. R. & Shipherd, J. C. (2016). Transforming a system: Improving patient-centered care for sexual and gender minority veterans. *LGBT Health*, *3*(3), 1–3.

Padula, W.V. Heru, S. & Campbell, J.D. (2016). Societal implications of health insurance coverage for medically necessary services in the U.S. transgender population: A cost-effectiveness analysis. *Journal of General Internal Medicine*, *31*(4), 394–401.

Ruben, M. A., Shipherd, J. C., AhnAllen, C. G., Sloan, C. A., Topor, D. Matza, A. (2017). Advancing LGBT healthcare policies and clinical care within a large academic medical center: A case study. *Journal of Homosexuality*. Epub ahead of print doi:10.1080/00918369.2017.1321386

Yehia, B. R., Calder, D., Flesch, J. D., Hirsh, R. L., Higginbotham, E., Tkacs, N., Crawford, B., & Fishman, N. (2015). Advancing LGBT health at an academic medical center: A case study. *LGBT Health*, *2*(4), 362–366.

References

Brown, G. R. (1988). Transsexuals in the military: Flight into hypermasculinity. *Archives of Sexual Behavior*, *17*, 527–537.

Cahill, S., & Makadon, H. (2014). Sexual orientation and gender identity data collection in clinical settings and in electronic health records: A key to ending LGBT health disparities. *LGBT Health*, *1*(1), 34–41.

Charness, M. (2011, May). *Management of Transgender Veteran Patients* [Patient Care Memorandum-11-046-LM]. Boston, MA: Department of Veterans Affairs, VA Boston Healthcare System.

Cochran, B. N. & Robohm, J. S. (2015). Integrating LGBT competencies into the multicultural curriculum of graduate psychology training programs. *Clinical Psychology: Science and Practice*, *22*(2), 119–126.

Cronk, T. M. (2016). *Transgender service members can now serve openly, Carter announces* [Press release]. Department of Defense. Retrieved from www.defense.gov/News/Article/Article/822235/transgender-service-members-can-now-serve-openly-carter-announces

Department of Veterans Affairs. (2015, May 11). *Rights and Responsibilities of VA Patients and Residents of Community Living Centers*. Retrieved from www.va.gov/health/rights/patientrights.asp

Department of Veterans Affairs. (2016a, November 15). *Medical Benefits Package*. Retrieved from www.va.gov/healthbenefits/access/medical_benefits_package.asp

Department of Veterans Affairs. (2016b, March 24). *Office of Health Equity: Healthcare Equality Index*. Retrieved from www.va.gov/healthequity/Healthcare_Equality_Index.asp

Department of Veterans Affairs. (2017a, May 8). *National Cemetery Administration*. Retrieved from www.cem.va.gov/

Department of Veterans Affairs. (2017b, May 8). *Veterans Benefits Administration*. Retrieved from www.benefits.va.gov/benefits

Department of Veterans Affairs. (2017c, May 2). *Veterans Health Administration*. Retrieved from www.va.gov/health

Elders, M. J., Brown, G. R., Coleman, E., Kolditz, T. A., & Steinman, A. M. (2014). Medical aspects of transgender military service. *Armed Forces & Society*, *41*(2), 1–22.

Gansler, L. L. (2005). *The mysterious Private Thompson: The double life of Sarah Emma Edmonds, Civil War soldier.* New York, NY: Free Press.

Gates, G. J., & Herman, J. L. (2014). *Transgender military service in the United States*. The Williams Institute. Retrieved from http://williamsinstitute.law.ucla.edu/wp-content/uploads/Transgender-Military-Service-May-2014.pdf

Kauth, M. R. & Shipherd, J. C. (2016). Transforming a system: Improving patient-centered care for sexual and gender minority veterans. *LGBT Health*, *3*(3), 1–3.

Kauth, M. R., Shipherd, J. C., Barrera, T. L., Ortigo, K., & Jones, K. R. (2016). Trainees' perceptions of the Veterans Health Administration interprofessional psychology fellowships in lesbian, gay, bisexual, and transgender health. *Training and Education in Professional Psychology*, *10*(3), 165.

Kauth, M. R., Shipherd, J. C., Lindsay, J. A., Kirsh, S., Knapp, H., & Matza, L. (2015) Teleconsultation and training of VA providers on transgender care: Implementation of a multisite hub system. *Telemedicine and e-Health*, *21*(22), 1–7.

Maguen, S., Shipherd, J. C. & Harris, H. N. (2005). Providing culturally sensitive care for transgendered patients. *Cognitive and Behavioral Practice*, *12*(4), 479–490.

Matza, A. R., Sloan, C. Kauth, M. R. (2015). Quality LGBT health education: A review of key reports and webinars. *Clinical Psychology: Science and Practice*, *22*(2), 127–144.

Padula, W. V., Heru, S. & Campbell, J. D. (2016). Societal implications of health insurance coverage for medically necessary services in the U.S. transgender population: A cost-effectiveness analysis. *Journal of General Internal Medicine*, *31*(4), 394–401.

Phillips, B. R., Shahoumian, T. A., & Backus, L. I. (2015). Surveyed enrollees in Veterans Affairs health care: How they differ for eligible veterans surveyed by BRFSS. *Military Medicine*, *180*(11), 1161–1169.

Shipherd, J. C., Kauth, M. R., Firek, A. F., Garcia, R., Mejia, S., Laski, S. J., Walden, B., Perez-Padilla, S., Lindsay, J. A., Brown, G., Roybal, L., Keo-Meier, C., Knapp, H., Johnson, L., Reese, R. L., & Byne, W. (2016). Interdisciplinary transgender veteran care: Training for Veterans Healthcare Administration providers. *Transgender Health*, *1*, 54–62.

Shipherd, J. C., Kauth, M. R., & Matza, A. (2016). Nationwide interdisciplinary e-consultation on transgender care in the Veterans Health Administration. *Telemedicine and E-health*, *22*(12), 1008–1012.

Index

Page numbers in italics refer to figures. Page numbers in bold refer to tables.